Patient Education:

YOU CAN DO IT!

GINGER KANZER-LEWIS, RN, BC, EdM, CDE

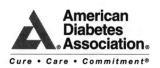

American Diabetes Association

Cure • Care • Commitment®

Director, Book Publishing, John Fedor; *Associate Director, Professional Books,* Christine B. Charlip; *Editor,* Joyce Raynor; *Associate Director, Book Production,* Peggy M. Rote; *Composition,* Circle Graphics; *Cover Design,* Mac Designs; *Printer,* Port City Press, Inc.

Printed in the United States of America
1 3 5 7 9 10 8 6 4 2

The suggestions and information contained in this publication are generally consistent with the Clinical Practice Recommendations and other policies of the American Diabetes Association, but they do not represent the policy or position of the Association or any of its boards or committees. Reasonable steps have been taken to ensure the accuracy of the information presented. However, the American Diabetes Association cannot ensure the safety or efficacy of any product or service described in this publication. Individuals are advised to consult a physician or other appropriate health care professional before undertaking any diet or exercise program or taking any medication referred to in this publication. Professionals must use and apply their own professional judgment, experience, and training and should not rely solely on the information contained in this publication before prescribing any diet, exercise, or medication. The American Diabetes Association—its officers, directors, employees, volunteers, and members—assumes no responsibility or liability for personal or other injury, loss, or damage that may result from the suggestions or information in this publication.

∞ The paper in this publication meets the requirements of the ANSI Standard Z39.48-1992 (permanence of paper).

ADA titles may be purchased for business or promotional use or for special sales. To purchase this book in large quantities, or for custom editions with your logo, contact Lee Romano Sequeira, Special Sales & Promotions, at the address below or at LRomano@diabetes.org, or call 703-299-2046.

American Diabetes Association
1701 North Beauregard Street
Alexandria, Virginia 22311

Library of Congress Cataloging-in-Publication Data

Kanzer-Lewis, Ginger, 1944-
    Patient education : you can do it! / Ginger Kanzer-Lewis.
        p. cm.
    Includes bibliographical references and index.
    ISBN 1-58040-162-7 (pbk. : alk. paper)
        1. Patient education. 2. Diabetes—Treatment. I. Title.

    R727.4.K36 2003
    616.4'62'0071—dc21

                                                   2003051854

Patient Education:

YOU CAN DO IT!

Dedication

This book is dedicated to all the people who have made my life and career a joy. It is dedicated to all the patients I ever taught and who taught me, to all the diabetes educators who ever worked for me and taught me what diabetes education is really about, and to my dears Liz Kennett, Gloria Coshigano, Virginia Rago, and Mary Lemeseveski. Can you imagine being a diabetes educator in my department? I am so grateful that they are my dearest friends to this day.

The book was possible because I met Betty Brackenridge and she got me involved with the American Association of Diabetes Educators (AADE) by telling me to put my money where my mouth is. She has been a mentor to me and so many others. The diabetes community is so lucky to have her.

I am full of gratitude and love for all the AADE presidents who dared me to go forward and pulled and pushed me up: Debbie Hinnen, Marilyn Graff, Jan Norman, Kathy Mulcahy, Chris Tobin, and for all the AADE staff who work so hard and put up with me. My sweet, dear Judy, what a year we had! I offer a prayer for all the presidents who will come after me and lead diabetes educators into the future, Kathy Berkowitz, Jane Kadahiro, Virginia Zamudio, Mary Austin, and those yet unnamed.

This book exists because of the love of my family, the real educators: my best friend and brother Mark and his wife Doctor Deena, my sister Sherry, and my children: Bill; Dawn, who did so much of the book for me; Kathy and Beth and their spouses; Jim; Ron; Jack; Donna; and especially my dear, own Glen who has been my joy always and his bride Helaina. It will be a remembrance for my grandchildren and great-grandchildren, and it is in memory of my parents Abraham and Pat, my brother Freddy, my sister Beth and for Bea and Sandy, who chose to be my parents.

I know there are lots of you not mentioned, and I ask your forgiveness for not thanking you here.

This book and I exist because of the Captain of my ship, my darling husband Jack. Safe waters always and all my love.

I love you all. Take care.

Ginger

Contents

Foreword

TEACHING: The earth doesn't move every time, but when it does, what a RUSH!
—Cameron Beatty

I consider myself remarkably lucky to have found my calling in health education. I get such a thrill when someone's face lights with insight. Or with determination. Or with pride and confidence. And that's still the case after 25 years of teaching in diabetes. That one field has remained new and challenging to me for one reason and it is this: The job of fostering learning is more about the people I serve than about the facts and processes I teach. The latter could get boring and stale if it were not for the utter diversity and challenge of the former.

The fact that you are reading this book suggests that you already share that thrill with me. Or perhaps you are looking for ways to bring it to your teaching. In either case, you are in for a treat.

One of the many gifts my calling has brought into my life is Ginger Kanzer-Lewis. Ginger, like me and most other teachers in the health field, is largely self-taught. We know our profession, be it nursing, dietetics, or some other baili-wick of medicine. And we have some body of knowledge to impart, be it diabetes, cardiac, asthma, or optimal health. But most of us became teachers either by edict or by choice, not by training. The result is one that Ginger and I have talked about many times—frequent frustration over both the task and the outcome.

This book is Ginger's offering to emerging and developing health facilitators. I know it is her hope that it will shorten the path from novice to technician to master, both for those entering the field and for those seeking further growth and skill.

> *Johnny:* I taught my dog Spike to whistle.
> *Lucy:* I don't hear him whistling!
> *Johnny:* I said I taught him. I didn't say he learned!

And make no mistake. We need all the help we can get! One of the main challenges in my experience lies in making sure that our teaching actually fosters learning. Teaching, after all, is not the end in itself, but simply a means to an end. Teaching takes place in the teacher. Learning is happening in the learner. Sometimes the gap between the two is huge.

Like Johnny teaching Spike to whistle, health educators are often teaching from their own needs rather than helping the patient learn what is truly needed and helpful. In this book, you will find a wealth of practical advice to help you sort the wheat from the chaff as you decide what to teach and how. The ultimate answer is "what the patient wants to learn." But there are tech-niques for engaging people and helping them find the meaning and importance of your message to them. Many of them are described in this book.

> *A good teacher is better than a spectacular teacher.*
> *Otherwise the teacher outshines the teachings.*
> —The Tao of Teaching

Learning is a lifetime task—or perhaps, more exactly, a lifetime privilege. Some have even suggested that ongoing learning is what makes a long life worth living. After all, those who learn keep a fresh outlook as they grow in skill and knowledge.

But the search for new knowledge and skills does not always grow out of choice. And that is the case with the people we serve as health educators. The need to learn or change has been thrust upon them by situations they would never have chosen: a heart attack, loss of hearing, worsening sight, or the diagnosis of a chronic condition such as asthma or diabetes.

Because of the reasons our patients come to us, we have a solemn obligation: to make sure that what we do makes a difference. As you read and practice the great tools presented here, keep in mind what your clients will say when you are done. Will it be, "He is a great teacher," or will it be, "I learned so much"?

> *It is the teacher's function to contrive conditions under which students learn.*
>
> —B.F. Skinner

I have had the privilege of watching Ginger teach a number of times over the years. And I always come away with new ideas to refresh my approach. I believe her genius lies in creating a rich environment for learning—one of relaxed fun, tinged with excitement, but always moving participants toward their own choices and growth. Much of her ease comes from experience and from utter familiarity with her subject. But part of it is technique as well. Scalpels do not make the surgeon, but she'd be up a creek without them.

In this book, she opens her toolbox to you. It is like having a master teacher looking over your shoulder. Enjoy!

Betty Brackenridge, MS, RD, CDE
Director, Professional Training
Diabetes Management & Training Centers, Inc.
Phoenix, Arizona

Preface

For over 35 years, I have been teaching health care professionals to teach. At first, they were nurses that I recruited to work in an inservice or staff development department. Fifteen years later, I found I could identify wonderful people and help develop diabetes educators and later patient educators. Little did I know that it would be a life-changing experience and ultimately lead me to the presidency of the American Association of Diabetes Educators.

This transition occurred because I turned down a job. I had interviewed for the position of Director of the Diabetes Teaching Nurses, as they were then called, at the Joslin Clinic in Boston. I had recently gotten my master's degree in Education at Harvard University, and there were very few nurses at that time with credentials in education. Adult Education was a new field and many people had not even heard about it as a specialty. I had also been in Staff Development and Education for 15 years and felt I had a pretty good handle on how to teach patients and how to get other professionals to teach patients. Evidently, Joslin agreed with me, as Denise Stevens offered me the position. I decided that the two-hour commute from New Hampshire was too long and regretfully turned her down. Two weeks later, she called and asked if I would teach an Adult and Patient Education portion for their four-day course for nurses and dietitians. I agreed. For the next 14 years, I taught the last day of that program. I called my section "Patient Education: Just Do It!" I have continued in my private consulting practice to teach that course and for 20 years have intended to put it all down on paper.

This book is a compilation of all the workshops, seminars, and classes I have taught during and since that time and is a practical guide to patient education. I believe it will give you much of the knowledge and skills you will need, tell you why you should teach patients, and tell you how people learn and how to turn them on. It will share with you practical knowledge and skills in developing classes, courses, and programs. It has taken me a lifetime to learn these skills, and I have wanted to give every bit of that information and passion to every educator I have worked with or met. These chapters will help you find easier, better, more fun, exciting, and stimulating ways to teach the same class you have been teaching or have been wanting to teach. There will be practical information that you can use immediately and take some of the fear and frustration that accompanies the new position of educator. For experienced educators, it will be a chance to reminisce, share, and laugh and perhaps learn a new trick or two or acquire a new idea or concept.

This is an opportunity to examine new ways to do the thing we love best. Teach patients.

This book includes all of the things I have learned from the best teachers in the world, patients and educators. I discovered that I learn every time I teach anyone anything and that is truly a gift. In the chapter on games and exercises, you will find out about my friends. I sent a call out to diabetes educators and asked them to share a game, exercise, or trick that they have learned in their personal practices. Many of them sent me their treasures and I have included them, with great joy, in my book. The reader will be the better for their knowledge and friendship. Enjoy.

I found a love of teaching early on in my career and to my great surprise a deep affinity for it. I remember, as a student nurse, an instructor telling me to consider going into nursing education. Evelyn Zalewski suggested it, and I laughed and told her I loved obstetrical nursing and that was where I would spend my career. She then told me something that I have shared with thousands of colleagues when trying to convince them to teach patients. "As long as someone remembers something you have said you are immortal." So many of my patients are immortal, for I remember something from everyone I have ever met.

My career has been, is, and will be an opportunity to do what I love best. I have been blessed!

1

Patient Education Defined

Here you will find not only my definition of patient education but also my approach to patient assessment.

er Webster's dictionary, a "patient" is "a person under Medical care" and to "educate" is "to supply with training or schooling: to supervise the mental or moral growth of." Although I cannot argue that most of our patients are under the care of a primary care provider, I believe that education cannot be explained with the term *training* or *schooling*.

I define patient education as a person with a health care need. To meet this need requires clear, concise information. My role is to give that person all the information they need to make decisions about what they will or will not do. This implies that the patient has some control over their lives. In the past, patients were told what to do by physicians and nurses and were expected to do as they were told. The "white coat syndrome" was the result of this authoritarian model that made no allowances for partnership with the patient or discussions of their life choices.

Anderson and Funnell[1] in their work on empowerment of patients talk about how for decades health care providers have taken over the role of manager in patient care and not allowed people to make decisions about their own lives. We also give them goals that are unachievable and get angry when they fail to achieve them. I have been in hundreds of patient care conferences where a group of professionals is judging the progress a patient is making or making decisions about future care *without the patient being present.* What is even worse is being in meetings where a family member is deciding what is best for his or her parent *with mama nowhere in sight.*

Bastable[2] is much more realistic when she defines patient education as a "process of assisting people to learn health-related behaviors in order to incorporate them into everyday life with the purpose of achieving the goal of optimal health and independence in self-care."[3] I am somewhat concerned with that broad statement. What is optimal? Can a patient who has suffered a CVA and right-sided hemiplegia realistically achieve optimal health and independence, or will they set and meet a specific, achievable goal?

You may notice that although much of the focus of this book is about people with diabetes, the concepts are applicable for all people with chronic diseases who have to live or manage some kind of disease process. Managing a cardiac condition is certainly as difficult and demanding as type 2 diabetes, and the parallels are very similar because both conditions may exist in the same person. Interestingly, the mother going home with a new baby may require a lot more instruction and information than a person who has just had hernia surgery.

The person going home from cardiac surgery needs as much education as any chronic disease patient. The statement then holds true that acute care patients may require as much or more infor-

---

[1] Anderson B, Funnell M: *The Art of Empowerment.* See References.

[2] Bastable S: *Nurse as Educator.* See References.

[3] Smith CE: Overview of patient education: opportunities and challenges for the twenty-first century. See References.

mation than the chronic disease patient but you have a shorter time to educate them, and they may require the skills and knowledge for a short time and then discard the information. I call that pulling the plug on unnecessary knowledge.

Here is an example: A patient has a tracheostomy after throat surgery. He is going home for two weeks and must care for his trach during that period of time. You teach him wound care, self-suctioning, aseptic technique, and how to assess for infection. Don't forget to teach him how to take his temperature and read a thermometer. You also, of course, make a referral for a visiting nurse to visit the patient and assist with the processes. Right? Right. Two weeks later the patient returns, the tracheostomy is closed, and the patient is breathing normally. Great. The patient no longer has to know or do some of those skills. There is nothing to suction. That plug is pulled, and they will very shortly forget that information. The mind doesn't often remember what is unnecessary. He will, however, always know how to take a temperature and read a thermometer because it is a skill that will be helpful to him for the rest of his life. Talking about surgical patients makes me think of something that has been bothering me for years.

It is very interesting to me that most patients who have open-heart surgery are given a red heart-shaped pillow. It is used for splinting the chest while coughing or moving and is quite helpful during the drive home from the hospital. If you had someone open your chest, you might want something soft to hold against it when you move. It then becomes logical that pillows, perhaps shaped like a uterus, would be given out to patients posthysterectomy. Would it be helpful to hold a pillow against your abdomen when you cough or drive home over potholes after you have abdominal surgery? If you handle postoperative patients, think about all aspects of their patient education and not just what is routine or has "always been done." After they recover from surgery, they will put the pillow aside—in essence, pull the plug—and never think of it again.

Several years ago, I was asked to see a patient in the critical care unit of my hospital who was recovering from open-heart surgery.

The patient had been diagnosed with type 2 diabetes and was having some difficulty adjusting to the management plan the nurse in the unit had developed for him. When I visited him and asked how long he had diabetes, he told me that his physician had diagnosed him the year before. He had been informed that he had a "mild case," and he and the doctor were going to concentrate on his cardiac condition first and then deal with his diabetes when his cardiac status was straightened out. After I finished my own cardiac arrest education, I assessed the patient to determine his health education needs. This person had to make major changes in his lifestyle to adjust to living with two major disease processes.

The educational concepts that educators use vary for each patient and are determined during the assessment process. Your first question must be, "What does this person need in order to safely live his life?"

Assessing Learning Needs

The first thing I find out is what the patient has been told and what he or she already knows. The easiest way to assess that is to ask.

What Has the Doctor Told You?

That is sometimes a difficult situation. If the physician was clear and concise and the patient was able to ask all the questions he or she needed to ask, we are in a much better place than we may be if the physician was vague or distracted.

In this case, I had to relate to a physician that people with diabetes have about four times greater risk of cardiac disease than people without diabetes and that diabetes and CVD interact. Sometimes, the education starts with the people who take care of patients.

Let's be clear about our medical colleagues. Most of the physicians I have worked with are incredibly committed and dedicated professionals. They work hard, long hours and are determined to give our patients the best care possible, in often difficult circumstances. There are never enough hours, people, or resources to meet the needs of their patients.

A family practice physician has to take care of patients with over 200 different diagnoses and keep up on the disease management changes that occur constantly in our field. It is amazing what they have to continually learn. I salute these colleagues with all my heart and partner with them in all kinds of venues and circumstances.

Some physicians do not take the time or have the energy or interest to keep current and do not rely on the colleagues available to them. They sometimes avoid taking the time to answer questions and expect patients to do as they are told without sufficient information or motivation.

It would be unethical and unprofessional for me to ever denigrate a colleague to a patient, and it often takes all my tack and diplomacy to get out of situations where my patients ask me why the doctor never told them this or that.

For example, I have a patient who is an active 45-year-old man. He has had diabetes for five years, and because he is a friend of mine, he came to me for help. He was told to watch what he ate and take two metformin tablets daily. When I asked him what kind of diabetes he had, he said the doctor told him that he did not have diabetes, just elevated sugars, and to watch himself. He was not told to test his blood or have glycated hemoglobin (A1C) tests done. He was not referred to an educator nor were goals set. It was not until three years later that the physician ordered quarterly A1C, after he apologized to the patient for not having them done earlier.

Diabetes educators have had to live with the terms "borderline diabetes" or "just a little bit of sugar" for years, and it is not acceptable. If the blood sugar is not normal, 90–110 mg/dl,[4] then the patient has impaired glucose tolerance. If it is above 126 mg/dl, the patient has diabetes. Short and simple. Calling these conditions

---

[4] American Diabetes Association: Standards of medical care for patients with diabetes mellitus (Position Statement). *Diabetes Care* 26 (Suppl. 1):S33–S50, 2003.

anything else is frustrating and often causes delay in the patient's ability to adapt to a long-term illness. It does nothing to assist the health educator to work more effectively with the patient in goal setting. The physician is doing the patient no favor by delaying a definitive diagnosis.

I have had to call a physician and ask for a diagnosis. One physician told me that he did not want to label the person as diabetic and put them through the stigma and insurance hassles. This is not acceptable in 2003.

What Does Having Diabetes Mean?

If the patient tells me that he has diabetes, I ask what he thinks that means and we go on from there. Some patients will say that they don't want to have diabetes. My answer is that I don't want to be short. It is a fact of life. I am short, and they have diabetes, and we will deal with it, and that is the pure truth.

How Do You Feel about Having Diabetes?

No one wants a disease that will not go away. It will be there for the rest of their lives. Diabetes takes no holidays, vacations, or days off. It is always there, and they will always have to deal with it. It is time-consuming and expensive and affects everything they do.

In Chapter 5, I talk about motivating patients. Before you can motivate them, you need to find out who they are and what they are about.

What Do You Know about Diabetes?

I learn a lot by asking this question. People have amazing ideas. They have often been educated by their favorite sources— neighbors, friends, relatives, pulp fiction, and tabloid newspapers. I try to keep aware of this "valid" information so I can deal with the many calls I receive when there is an article published telling people that islet cells can now be eaten to cure diabetes. Just in case you are curious, I just made that up! Our ability to unteach myths and find the realities for patients is often the most important thing we do.

This does not only apply to people with diabetes. People are happy to get information from nonprofessionals because it is never threatening or fatal. If you don't like what your neighbor tells you, go to another neighbor. This tactic often delays care or treatment and can be life-threatening. We need to create an environment that is neither frightening nor intimidating that allows the patient to ask questions without a fear of being thought stupid or naïve. Give the patient permission to disagree with you or argue about a concept. If you tell patients that they have the final say on their own life, then you are assuring them that you respect them as people.

The rest of the assessment is the process we utilize in health care constantly. In nursing, we call it "The Nursing Process," but most health professionals follow a close proximity. Who is this patient as a person? What are her psychosocial needs? Does she have a support structure? Is there a significant other to help her through the learning process? Are there barriers to learning? Can she afford to live with this disease? What parts of the health care system will she utilize? What referrals will she require? Which members of the health care team are needed at this time or will be required at a later date?

The data you collect from the patient will give you a clear picture of this patient and how you can help him or her achieve his or her goals and objectives.

Collecting the physical data gives us a clear picture of what is happening to this patient and what changes need to be made in his or her physical picture overall. Part of this may be determining what data need to be collected in order to make clear decisions about treatments. One or two blood tests are not going to give me all the information I need to help the patient learn meal planning and make lifestyle changes. I cannot do pattern management without a pattern to analyze.

Compare this to an educational assessment. What does the person have to know, how does he learn, how ready is he to learn, and what are the barriers? In Chapter 4 on the Do-Know-Deficit, I will take you through the entire process of assessing learning needs.

Once you have assessed learning needs, you develop an education plan for that individual. The plan is developed in conjunction with the patient and, if possible, the significant other. Be realistic. What does this person need to know? There are three considerations: needs to know, wants to know, and nice to know.

The "needs to know" are the essential components. These are the survival skills, the basic things a patient needs to know to go home safely. In diabetes, I call them the four M's: medication, meal planning, monitoring, and motivation. The patient needs this knowledge to leave your care safely.

The "wants to know" are the things that patients ask about. They may not be the most important things to you, but if the patient asks about something and you close the subject or shut them out, they will not hear anything else you say. For example, most of us divide our classes into several sessions. Perhaps the first class is "what is diabetes?" The second class is meal planning, and the third session is medications. Sound familiar?

Perhaps the first night you notice a patient looking very nervous and fidgety. When you go over the outline for the programs, the patient states that he was told he has to start on insulin "shots" next week and is worried about that. If you close him off by telling him that the subject will be covered in the medication class, three days later, he will be completely turned off. He may not even return for the rest of the classes and will absolutely not hear anything you say for the rest of the first class.

This is a teachable moment. These are so exciting, and when they occur, you have the best opportunity to get through to patients. They want to know something, so they have opened their minds to information and concepts. This is a wonderful chance to really get through to them and, if you miss that moment, you may never get it again. You can tell them that the subject will be covered later on, but that if they are really concerned you will discuss it with them after the class. That will show your concern but also let them know that the entire class is not there to meet their specific needs. In a large class, we have to create teachable moments. It is harder and a lot of work. I strive to create an atmosphere where people want to listen to me and learn. When I lead an all-day workshop, I ask an audience to give me the first two hours, and if I am not getting through to them, they have my permission to leave and we will give them back their money. I do not hold hostages!

Finally, there are the "nice to knows." These are things that may be interesting and fun but no one needs them to survive. I remember teaching a section on "how to travel with insulin." It was part of my medication class and was taught regularly. It was a long time before I realized that most of the people in my class had never been out of Nashua, New Hampshire, let alone to the Grand Canyon in 110° heat. Teach what the people need, not what you enjoy. You may have a great time in your favorite class, but it may be useless to your patients.

Patient educating can be exciting, inspiring, motivating, and wonderful. It can also be frustrating, exhausting, demanding, and frightening. It will be what you make it.

2

Why Do Patient Education?

Here are my thoughts on the importance of patient education and how to approach the legal, moral, ethical, and professional issues of patient education.

In these times of nursing shortages and time constraints created by managed care companies, how dare I suggest that you need to educate patients? When health care providers of all disciplines are being asked to do more with less each day, how can patient education really be done?

When only the most acutely ill are allowed to be admitted as inpatients in hospitals and the outpatient departments are overflowing with needy people, when patients may wait three or four months to get appointments for outpatient clinics and the waiting list is continually growing, how dare I insist that patients have a right to be taught?

There are critical issues to be addressed. Why should patients be taught at all?

It Is the Legal Thing to Do

Think about it. If you are a nurse, this situation will ring true: All of us have given a patient a drug that requires that you take a pulse before administration of that medication. We would never consider giving that one pill without personally taking a pulse. Some of us even take apical radial pulses. An example would be a digitalis tablet. Now think about this. Have you handed a patient a prescription for 100 digitalis tablets and not asked him whether he knew how to take a pulse? Have you asked him to show you how to take a pulse and validated that he was doing it correctly? You would not give the patient one pill without taking that pulse, and yet you would send the patient home with a lethal dose of medication without making sure he had instructions to keep him safe?

I can think of another example: A patient has a simple fracture and cast but requires crutches for non–weight-bearing walking. If the patient is not taught to walk correctly with the crutches and falls, refracturing the leg, you are legally responsible. These patients trust you to administer medications, teach them treatments, and make sure they are leaving the facility no worse than when they entered.

My cousin had a total hip replacement while in his early 40s. He left the hospital and was told to avoid soft seats and make sure to always sit on a hard surface. He went home and sat on a solid leather sofa that happened to be too low. He dislodged his hip and had to be returned to the hospital that day for additional surgery. No one had said anything about chair height.

My son went to college in Florida and worked part-time as a lifeguard. He developed a sore throat and went to the infirmary for care. The physician prescribed tetracycline. Think about that: tetracycline—Florida—lifeguard. Every person who administers that drug knows to tell the person to stay out of the sun. The sun can cause a severe burn to *that* person on *that* drug. Would you have wanted to be the nurse on the other end of the phone when I called to question the care?

It Is the Moral Thing to Do

We have a responsibility to advocate for our patients and protect them from any harm, especially from our colleagues and us. People in our care are entitled to know that we will do right by them. We will be honest and protect them whenever we can. Each of us has stepped in when circumstance put us in the position of patient advocate. I have had to step into a code situation where CPR is being done incorrectly and take over. If someone is tactfully told to let me, a CPR Instructor Trainer, handle it and refuses, I need to be more assertive and deal with the consequences later on.

I have spoken to many people with diabetes, and they come to us with a lot of "garbage" about the health care industry. Some of them have been dealt with very badly and incorrectly by professionals and come to us with fear, concern, and a history of poor care. We often have to prove that we are competent and capable. They don't know who we are. Are you wonderful? Are you the best you can be? Did you graduate at the top of your class or at the bottom? They are entrusting themselves to people whom they did not know an hour earlier and giving them major decision-making power over their lives.

That is a lot of responsibility. We are the only professionals responsible for the intimate care of strangers. We ask them to do all kinds of things and tell us about their most personal issues, and we are therefore responsible not to betray that trust. In Chapter 14 on the patient's perspective, I give you actual examples of the poor health care experiences of people I have met or with whom I have worked.

It Is the Ethical Thing to Do

Ethics are the guiding principles of human behavior. How do we behave toward people? Are they important human beings who have needs and specific concerns? I have a cartoon in my office of a patient sitting up in bed, talking to his wife. He tells her that yesterday he was the chairman of the board and today he is the gallbladder in 254. Are your patients people, or just patients? People have expectations about us, and unfortunately, many of them have been disappointed in the past. We cannot send people out of our care unprepared for self-care or without turning them over to another appropriate health care professional.

It Is the Professional Thing to Do

The Nurse Practice Act of each state says that the registered nurse will do patient education. If you examine the expectations of each of the other professionals, dietitians, physicians, social workers, and physical therapists, they are expected to do the same. You must adhere to these legal expectations of your profession. It does not say, do it when you have the time. Nowhere is it written that only educators are held accountable.

The Joint Commission for Accreditation of Healthcare Organizations, JCAHO, says that all patients are entitled to patient education and hold health care facilities accountable for having policies and procedures that explain how this is done and by whom. It is a wonderful mandate for us and really helps convince people that what we do is important and of value.

There is no need for patient education to be a burden. There is no expectation for unit personnel, be they nurses, dietitians, or pharmacists, to conduct formal classes on the units. If you give patients a medication, teach them about it. If you discuss a special "diet" with patients, talk to them about meal planning at home. If you change a dressing, explain the follow-up care required at home. This should become part of all care for people in any health care facility. I know that patients are taught when we get a free minute, extra staff, or a lapse in urgent activity. Everything else gets caught up in the routines of our day and is put aside. It can be even worse in a clinic where patients are in and out so quickly that you miss them and the opportunities to teach them. Can patients use waiting room time more effectively? Can a video be shown in the area to reinforce your teaching? Can an awareness tape on smoking cessation be part of the "background noise" in the clinic area? Maybe they will find themselves watching despite feeling bored. The TV is often on in waiting areas, so show something educational.

I met a pharmacist once who works in a large hospital in Chicago and was a participant in my patient education workshop. He raised his hand at this point in the discussion and told me that he teaches people every day and was indeed the "discharge pharmacist." When I asked for clarification, he explained that he had an office at the front door of the hospital and that every patient would stop at his office on the way out, where he would teach them about their medications. Picture this: the patient is on his way out, he has his coat on and his luggage in hand, and his wife is waiting outside with the car or a cab with the meter running. This is when he is taught about an important medication.

I suggested that he get out of his office and go to the units to teach the patients while they would be interested in hearing from him. I also asked him how often he did medication reviews and updates for the staff members on the units who were administering medications. People do not do things outside of their comfort zone, and if the staff is unsure or uncertain about something, they certainly will not teach about that subject.

3

The Adult Learner

Let's discuss my favorite subject:
adult education.

Malcolm Knowles is considered the father of the adult education movement in the United States. He was an amazing man, and in his book *The Adult Learner: A Neglected Species,*[5] he makes an incredible statement. He wrote, "We know more about how animals (especially rodents and pigeons) learn than how children learn: and we know more about how children learn than how adults learn." He wrote this over 30 years ago, and we have learned a great deal during that period of time, but it remains amazing to me that we find educators everywhere who are still treating adult people as slightly moronic 6-year-olds.

He said that the reason that adults have difficulty learning is that they are taught by people who are either

---

[5] Knowles M: *The Adult Learner: A Neglected Species.* Houston, TX, Gulf Publishing, 1973.

experts in their subjects and don't know how to teach or by
teachers who were trained to teach children and not adults.

Have you ever been a college student who was treated as if you
were a child? Did you resent it? I will give you an example. I am
a diploma graduate in nursing, so I had to go back to college and
take the same courses that I took in nursing school. It had been
decided that nurses who were educated off college campuses
would not receive academic credit for those courses, so I was
taking anatomy and physiology again, and I am skinning a cat
10 years after I skinned the first one. Now, we get to final examination time, and I am well prepared. I was sure that "the eye"
would be on the final exam because the professor had spent six
weeks on the eye and two weeks on the heart. I prepared well and
if given a model of the eye, or a diagram, could accurately identify
all of the components. Great. I need an A because I am a nurse
and compulsive. The night of the exam arrives, and I open the
exam, and it says, "draw and label a diagram of the eye." I raise my
hand and the professor comes over for my question. I stated my
concern that I do not draw well, and if I draw an eye, he will not
recognize the components and will deduct points. He said to just
draw an eye. I told him that this was not an art class and if he gave
me a diagram I would label it absolutely accurately. He said just
draw it, and you will not lose points. I wrote on my paper, "I will
not accept any deduction in points because of this poor art work.
This is not an art class." I had him sign it. I got an A on my eye.

Think about what you ask patients to do, how you ask them to
do it, and their treatment as adults.

Andragogy means adult education, versus pedagogy, or the
teaching of children. It stems from the Greek word *aner*, meaning
man as distinguished from boy, and was originally used by the
educators in Yugoslavia. It is rarely found in dictionaries, which
drives many of my colleagues crazy when they try to validate adult
education methodology.

I started my first diabetes education program in 1972 when I
was Director of Staff Development in a hospital in New Hampshire. The nursing staff came to me for help with inpatients who

had been diagnosed with diabetes. We had few materials in those days to help us teach patients. There was a tear sheet on oral medications and a small booklet from Eli Lilly and Company about insulin. Patient education was a new idea in the Northeast, and pioneers like the Joslin Diabetes Center were doing groundbreaking work. If you were not in the "diabetes world," you really did not know what was happening in other parts of the country, and many of us were operating in the dark.

I started teaching patients with handmade materials, and it took me over a year to develop a manual to give to "diabetic patients." Before you think I was an idiot, please remember that I was operating in the adult education world 10 years before I finally enrolled in Harvard for a master's degree in Education. Dr. Knowles had not even written his book on adult education. I took my beautiful new manual to a newly diagnosed patient one day and told her to read the book and she would know everything about diabetes. No assessment, or even a conversation. I returned the next day and asked her what she had learned. She responded, in French, that she could not read or speak English. I had given her this beautiful book, and it was worth nothing. I had not taken the time to find out who this woman was and what she needed from me.

Let's think about the adult learner. Adults will learn what they want to learn, when they want to learn it, and your job is to facilitate that learning experience. We are talking about changing behaviors. Change is always frightening, and when you are talking about life and death issues, it can be so frightening that it is paralyzing.

When dealing with adults, the terms *relevant* and *validating* are so important. The first rule of adult education is: Don't teach *junk*! If I don't need to know it and it will not impact my life, do not teach it to me. Adults do not have time in their lives and minds for unnecessary information. Your job is to find out what is relevant to each individual and give him or her that information.

Consider adult education a partnership with another individual who is on an equal plane with you. He may have less, or more, education than you have, but he brings to the partnership life-long learning experience that may help or hinder the learning process. He may be an expert in another field and need more scientific data from you than most people require. Your assessment will help you determine his learning needs. I give my patients permission to disagree with me on the importance of certain actions that I expect from people with diabetes.

Here is an example on the topic of exercise. I encourage every person to increase their physical activity level when diagnosed with diabetes, but I have to be realistic. Here is a person, perhaps 55 years of age, who has never done physical activity as an adult. It is unreasonable for me to expect her to join a gym and start being active just because I suggest it. I need to convince her of the need for more movement and help her find a reasonable activity. I hate to exercise, but I really love to dance. Does that make sense? I actually state that to my patients, and we talk about alternatives. Adults need to analyze information and synthesize it with their lifestyle.

Several years ago, my husband Jack went to the doctor after being diagnosed with type 2 diabetes. My husband is an interesting man. He is the biggest pain in the neck I ever met but an amazing man. You need to know that we live on a boat in the Florida Keys, and we worked hard all our lives to be able to do this. Jack had emergency angioplasty, and I told him in the recovery room that he was fine and that I had called the boat dealer and ordered the boat we had been debating about when the doctor told me that he was going to be fine. After such a close call, I was not going to chance waiting any longer to buy the boat. Now, that boat means everything to Jack. Our doctor told him that he now had to lose 50 pounds and start exercising. Jack said "no." The doctor repeated that it is essential that he lose 50 pounds and exercise. Jack asked the doctor, a great friend of ours who has kept us both alive longer than we ever expected, what part of the word "no" did he not understand. Then the doctor said, "You know, Jack, if you don't take care of yourself, you're going to drop dead, and I know three guys who are perfect for Ginger." Jack said, "Great, she'll be comfortable and fine." I am sitting there with smoke coming out of my ears, but I didn't say a word until we got in the car. Then I clued him in. "If you don't care who is going to be sleeping with me, I want you to think about who is going to be driving your boat." He lost 30 pounds and started walking two miles a day. His A1C is 6%, and he will probably outlive me. The message is to talk to adults about what is important to them. Read Chapter 6 on motivation.

Oermann[6] and Bell[7] discuss some important variables in adult education:

- readiness to learn
- past experiences
- health status
- environmental stimuli
- anxiety level
- developmental stage
- practice session length

Learning does not exist in a vacuum. Adults seldom live in this world completely alone, and their environment and support system often is the main determinant of whether the patient succeeds or fails in his or her learning experience.

We need to make what we do relevant to them and purposeful in their lives. It upsets me terribly when a patient says that he keeps a log of his daily blood sugars and takes them to his doctor at each visit but it is never looked at or used for pattern management. How can we ask patients to do things that are meaningless?

Here is an example of a patient problem. Jack (another Jack) was in my outpatient class and attended with his wife. He is a charming, delightful man who just happens to look just like Santa Claus, beard and all. We get to the point in the class where the pharmacist is teaching the class, and she explains that you pick up the insulin bottle and roll it gently because you don't want to damage the insulin or get bubbles in the bottle. Jack states that he

[6] Oermann MH: Psychomotor skill development. *J Contin Educ Nurs* 21:202–204, 1990.

[7] Bell ML: Learning a complex nursing skill: student anxiety and the effect of preclinical skill evaluation. *J Nurs Educ* 30:222–226, 1991.

shakes his insulin all the time. This gentleman has been in our hospital system for two years. He has not been to class before but he has been in ICU, the outpatient medical clinic, the emergency room, and on the medical surgical units during the previous two years. I ask him, "Do you mean you leave the bubbles in? How do you get them out before you inject yourself?" He says he draws the insulin up and always gets bubbles and just injects them into his abdomen. I asked him to show me his abdomen, and he is covered with bubbles under his skin: crepitus. The man was injecting the insulin with "bubbles" into his skin. It now occurs to me why his blood sugar is out of control: He never gets the same dose of insulin. Every injection is different depending on how much air is in the syringe. My question is for the health care providers who cared for him in the previous two years. Who validated that this man was capable of giving himself injections?

So, we taught Jack the proper technique and validated that he could do it correctly. At this point, I had major concerns and arranged for Jack to call me every day for the next week with his blood sugars. I wanted to make sure that he avoids hypoglycemia, as he is now getting the correct dose of insulin.

I also had to perform a quality improvement review and investigate the root causes of this major problem. Why was the staff giving the patients their injections instead of supervising the patients' self-administration? The reply was ludicrous: they knew that diabetics had to give their shots at home so they did it for them in the hospital to give them a rest. They eat at home too but we don't just feed everyone in the hospital to give them a rest.

It is not valuable for health care providers to do tasks for patients that the patients need to learn to do for themselves. Adults need to practice psychomotor skills in front of people who can validate the correctness of the task before they practice it incorrectly at home.

My granddaughter broke her leg, and they told her "no bathing or swimming this month." It was July, and she was upset and angry. They showed her how to wrap her cast, which enabled her to shower, but it was not good enough for Tara. She was a teenager

THE ADULT LEARNER 21

at the time and ticked off that her summer was being ruined. She had been told not to swim or bathe, but no one had said anything about not lying on a lawn chair and holding the garden hose over her head to cool off on a hot summer day. The cast started to smell, and when we noticed green things starting to grow out of the cast, it was time for a visit to the orthopedic specialist for a cast change. We had not explained the ramifications or alternatives; we just told her what to do and expected her to follow orders. Adults do not follow orders well. I really have no right to insinuate that teenagers are adult people, but I try.

You need to ask people what they are willing to do to survive. How hard are they willing to work, and what are they willing to learn? If we teach them survival skills, they do much better than if we ask them to learn everything about diabetes immediately. A great little book was developed by the Metropolitan New York Association of Diabetes Educators[8] that really helps define what people with diabetes need to learn.

I have had patients tell me that they are not ready for this process. They cannot handle the stress, and they are frightened or in denial. The most difficult thing I ever wrote in a chart is that the patient is uneducable. I would not write that now. Instead, I might say that the person is uneducable at this time and define the barriers. I would then make a referral to another health care provider in the community and notify the primary care physician of the problems and obstacles. I would also make sure to contact the patient in the future and check on his or her state of mind and motivational status.

When I worked in the hospital, I was notified if one of my patients arrived in the emergency department in crisis. There might be a person with a blood sugar of 500 or 700 mg/dl. And I would ask the person, "Why is your blood sugar so high?" Everyone would be running around doing diagnostic tests, CAT scans,

---

[8] Metropolitan New York Association of Diabetes Educators: *Guide to Teaching Diabetes Survival Skills.* Chicago, IL, American Association of Diabetes Educators, 1995.

blood work, and blood cultures, and I am talking to the person. There are only a few reasons that a blood sugar would be that high. The person did not take her medications, she ate everything in sight, she has an infection, or something unusual is going on in her life. So I ask them. In one episode, the person went to a wedding and drank everything available. His daughter was getting married, and he decided to take the day off from being a diabetic. He never got to eat all day, but everyone gave him a drink to celebrate. Sounds like fun to me but not too clever. Hyper- or hypoglycemia is not a fun experience.

The most important part of adult learning is accurate, clear, concise communication. This is the hardest thing we do as adults, and it is not something we learn in school. Unless you chose a communication course in college, it is never part of your academic life. Yet, all teaching is communication.

Communication is the act of transferring an idea or message, for the purpose of eliciting a response. Most of us just talk. We send words and ideas into the atmosphere and hope that someone will catch the message out there and pay attention.

To say that you are communicating assumes that what you are saying requires some response. The response does not have to be verbal. A person can nod or just change his or her affect, and you know that he or she has received the message. One-way communication is so often the way people are taught. Think about a huge lecture hall where students sit, listen to the professor, and take notes. The only way teachers find out if the message got through is at the time of final exams when a test score is supposed to tell them how successfully they were educating. That may be acceptable, but I cannot imagine anyone accepting it as an adult education method. Adults need an opportunity to analyze information and adapt it to their own lives.

Communication can be divided into two sections: verbal and nonverbal.

Verbal communication includes anything that uses language or words. It can be spoken, written, or sung. English is the hardest

Communication Methods

Verbal
- Spoken
- Written
- Sung

Nonverbal
- Facial expressions
- Posture
- Gestures

- Body movement
- Tone or voice pitch
- Speed of speech

language of all because there are so many definitions for simple words. Here's an example of a simple word that can mean many things.

Fast can mean speed, quick, hurry. It can also mean not move at all as in hold fast.

Then we can talk about fasting—not eating. Does that mean not eating at all, NPO? Nothing at all? We tell a patient that he or she is fasting for blood work, but what does that mean? I told my daughter that she was fasting for surgery and was NPO. She asked what NPO meant, and I replied that NPO stands for nothing by mouth. N, nothing, P . . . by? O is mouth? I responded that it was Latin, *noti per os*, and she asked when had she learned Latin? Take it further. To Catholics, fasting means no meat on Friday or abstaining from a large meal on Good Friday. To Jews, it means nothing to eat or drink on Yom Kippur. You tell a person to fast for blood work, and he or she may eat everything but meat. You can think of another framework: How about the old terminology, a fast woman? In Jamaica, fast means sly and nosy.

My daughter was right. If your patients don't understand you, what did you tell them? If they do not do as you asked, what did you ask them to do?

I am not asking you to sing to people, but it can be a very useful tool when dealing with an illiterate person or a child who has difficulty remembering a sequence of activities.

A great example is the McDonald's jingle telling us how to make a Big Mac. I bet you know the song.

I have changed the words of an old song to help children remember how to give insulin injections. Think of the old tune "Ball in the Jack." Here it is translated:

First you roll the insulin round and round
Then you put the needle in and make the bubble go down
Turn the bottle over pull the plunger out again
And then you rub and you rub and you rub your skin
Put the needle in, push the plunger down, pull the needle out,
   rub it round and round
Write it down in your little book
And that's what I call insulin Jack

If I tell you that I bought my kid a bike, what do I mean? A two-wheeler bicycle? My youngest is thirty-three. A motorcycle? If I told you I bought my granddaughter a bike, would you think a tricycle? She is a grown woman and a nurse.

When you tell people to do something, you need to validate the message. How can that be done without insulting people? There is a hidden word in the English language. {Dummy!}

We don't say it out loud, but it is clear and loud. You say to people, "And you know how to take this medication, don't you?" {Dummy} "You understand what I mean, don't you?" {Dummy} And people are afraid to tell you they don't understand.

The first thing I learned was that adults are never wrong. They cannot handle being told they are wrong. They will not hear another word you say after that, because they will be so busy defending themselves and what they know. We have to take the word *dummy* out of conversations with patients. Think about what women say to their husbands: "Are you really going to wear that shirt with that tie?" {Dummy!}

When you say to a person, this is what I want you to do, do you understand? They will always tell you "yes." Usually they shake their heads affirmatively. I call this the bobbing head syndrome— like the little dogs in the back of the car. It is demeaning for many people to admit that they do not understand what you mean.

How can you ask the same question and leave out the dummy? How about using validation techniques? Say to the patient, "Tell me what you are going to do when your blood sugar is below 60? I just want to make sure that I told it to you correctly." In this instance, you take the responsibility for the communication experience. If they misheard or misunderstood, you are willing to assume (they think) that you communicated the message poorly.

Then, there are the **nonverbal** communication components:

- body language
- facial expressions
- posture
- gestures
- body movement
- tone or pitch of voice
- speed of speech

Each of these should be considered when you evaluate your teaching techniques and communication methods.

How do you move around people? Are you too close or too far? Do you overwhelm them with grand gestures? Do you watch people's faces when you step over the line into their personal space?

Can they understand your fast talking style? I am from New York and have to deliberately slow down when I speak in different parts of the country or overseas. If you overwhelm people, they will be watching you instead of listening to what you are saying.

We all know people who never do as you ask. What did you really ask them to do? If you think this validation takes too much time, think about how much time you spend redoing or reteaching something because the other person did not understand and you did not take the time to validate.

How do people learn? This may be one of the most valuable tools I give you.

People remember 10% of what they read. That's all. We send memos out to the world, and no one remembers what they said. They are usually on white paper with small, black writing. If you send out messages, print them on colored paper with pictures and large type. If you are giving people manuals, they must be

Learner's Ability to Retain Information

- 10% of what is read
- 26% of what is heard
- 30% of what is seen
- 50% of what is seen and heard
- 70% of what is said as they talk
- 90% of what is said as they do something

considered an adjunct to education and not a substitution for education.

People remember 26% of what they hear. If you are just lecturing to people, they will remember only a quarter of what you are saying. Don't just talk at people.

People remember 30% of what they see. If you show me how to test my blood, and I just watch you, I will only remember a third of what I saw—not really good percentages when I am doing something that might be lifesaving.

People remember 50% of what they see and hear. When we don't know what to teach, we show movies. Now we use videotapes, a movie in a box. I cannot ask questions, and the movies do not validate what I have learned. Another disappointment.

People remember 70% of what they say. If I explain something to you, I retain 70% of that knowledge. When I am preparing for an exam, if I find people to teach the subject to, I have a better chance of remembering that data because I said it myself.

The best number is the last. People remember 90% of what they say as they do something. If I test my blood or change my dressing and explain what I am doing as I actually do it, I have 90% retention.

These are still not very good percentages, so we have to add them together. If I show and tell you something, it's 50%, then I have you tell me what you are going to do, that adds 70%. Then I have you do it and tell me what you are doing, which adds 90%. Now I give you a film to take home, add 50%, and I give you a manual, 10%. The total is now up to 270%. Now we are on the right path. Data have shown that people forget 50% of what they have learned from their physician by the time they reach the car in the parking lot. Even if we divide 270% in half we are still dealing with a 135% retention in learning. That's really pretty good.

I have a suggestion. Find a day when your hair looks really good and you don't feel fat. Have someone tape your class and make copies of the tape for your patient. If you give people a commercial tape, they may or may not look at it. If you send a tape of you to the patient's home, it is a different situation completely. The person takes it home and says to his daughter, "Come watch this, it's my teacher." They may watch it together and then he may show it to a friend or neighbor. You have a much better chance of him wanting to watch your tape than one showing a complete stranger teaching. You can reduce the cost of doing this by having patients bring you blank tapes in order to get their copy. Ask your kids to make the copies for you. They are much better at it then you are, anyhow.

Many of your patients will have English as a second language. Their English may not contain idioms or slang expressions that you include in your vocabulary. Watch for body language to tell you whether the person is on your wavelength.

Cultural issues become very important in patient education. People from Mediterranean countries are very passionate. They can handle grandiose gestures and analogies. If you are dealing with men from South America, there is a macho issue to consider with your communication. They might not be happy getting instructions from a female if they think you are talking down to them or giving them orders. When I lectured to Japanese physicians in Mexico City, I was told not to tell any jokes in my presentation and be very formal in addressing the doctors. It was very difficult for me to be straight when lecturing. It was very stressful for me but a wonderful learning experience.

We need to get everyone in this patient's health care community speaking the same language, i.e., using the same terminology when talking about the disease process. It is confusing for people to hear one health care provider say they have type 2 diabetes and have another tell them they have non-insulin-dependent diabetes mellitus, especially if they are taking insulin injections. Be consistent.

4

The Do-Know-Deficit

Let's look at transferring adult education knowledge into adult education methodology.

The first step in developing any program is to decide what topic you want to teach. To do that, you need to identify what the learner has to do. Before you decide that focusing only on what he or she has to do is pedagogical or childish, I ask you to go forward with a little trust.

Let's start with something completely out of the realm of diabetes and work with a new mother on the OB unit. What does a new, inexperienced mother have to do for a new baby?

List of "do's" for a new mother:

- bathe the baby
- feed the baby
- change a diaper
- wash the baby's hair
- cord care
- respond to baby's cries
- comfort the baby
- give the baby vitamins or medication
- travel safely with the baby

- clean the eyes
- burp the baby
- dress the baby
- take a temperature
- bond with the baby
- put the baby in a car seat
- put together a baby bag
- buy clothes for the baby
- select appropriate toys for the baby

I am sure you might come up with a few additional things! Now let's select one item from the list and identify everything the mother has to "know" in order to "do" that thing. How about "changing the baby"?

- select the correct size diaper
- buy the diapers
- select cloth or disposable
- if cloth:
  - where to buy
  - how many
  - what size
  - Velcro or pins
  - plastic pants
  - cost
  - how to put them on
  - how to fold them when clean
  - where to keep the pins
  - where to keep the dirty diapers
- how to flush full diapers
- If disposable:
  - what size
  - boy or girl diapers
  - how many
  - where to buy
  - how to save money with coupons
  - how to apply
  - how to remove when full
  - where to store
  - how to dispose of them
  - use a Diaper Genie?

Once you have the diapers:

- how to remove the diaper
- how to clean the baby
- wipes
- soap and water
- powder or lotion
- diaper rash
- creams and ointments
- how to apply creams and ointments
- which ointments
- where to change the baby
- how to travel with diapers

Now that you have identified all the "knows," there is a content list for your class. Before you do the curriculum development, however, there is the most important step. Because you are working with adults, identify what they already know. How do you do that? You ask them!

Show them the list and ask them what they already know and because you are responsible for the safety of that little baby, validate! If they say they are only going to use disposable diapers, do not teach them from the list on cloth diapers. That does not free you from developing the curriculum on cloth diapers; after all, the next mother may make that choice and you will want to have that ready.

Now that you know what they have to do, you know what they have to know to do it, and what they already know . . . teach the deficit!

Remember, do not teach adults junk. Do not teach me what I do not need to live my life or what I already know. I do not have the time or energy to learn unnecessary information.

Let's do a practical exercise for a person with diabetes. What does he or she need to do?

List of do's for a person with diabetes:

- manage a meal plan
- take oral medications
- inject insulin
- test blood
- foot care
- exercise
- follow-up medical visits
- have eye exams
- record data
- watch blood pressure
- check cholesterol
- travel with medications
- monitor weight

We are ready to select one of the do's to create the "know" list. Let's select "inject insulin." To inject insulin, the person will have to know:

- which insulin to take
- what dose at what time
- how to buy insulin
- where to buy insulin
- how to buy syringes
- where to buy syringes
- carrying syringes when traveling
- the actions of insulin
- cost
- expiration dates
- the side effects
- how to recognize hypoglycemia
- how to treat hypoglycemia
- how to inject glycogen
- how to use food to deal with hypoglycemia
- the simple sugars for treatment
- how to select injection sites
- absorption rates at injection sites
- how to select a syringe
- how to draw insulin into a syringe
- how to remove air from syringes
- how to put a needle into skin
- how to prepare the skin
- aseptic technique
- how to dispose of syringes
- how to rotate sites
- how to document the injection administration

Now you are ready to check with the patient about his or her knowledge, skill, attitudes, and previous experience administering insulin. The patient looks at the list and identifies what he or she already knows; you validate and then teach the deficit! Simple. It seems to make sense and prepares you for the next step, which is to prepare the lesson plan.

Think about the simplicity of this process. If you were doing something as simple as teaching a nursing assistant to make a bed, it would be very simple and take no time at all to develop the lesson plan. Realistically, it does take time and effort to develop the Do-Know-Deficit for everything you teach, but you really only have to do it once.

This is a very simple process, and I have been using it since 1980. I have found it fun and often ask a colleague to brainstorm the components of the do's and know's. Think about the lists above. Can you add to them and see what I may have missed? I did this class for a group of dietitians once, and the topic they chose was making chicken gravy. The list was so long and in-depth that they went all the way back to the barnyard and had me chasing the chicken. Have fun!

Let me give you a template.

1. What does the person have to DO?

   _____

   _____

   _____

   _____

2. What does the person have to KNOW in order to DO that?

   _____

   _____

   _____

   _____

3. What does the person already KNOW? Cross those objects off the list. (Only after you identify, validate, and document that he or she really knows each one.)

   _____

   _____

   _____

   _____

4. Teach the DEFICIT (This is your class content.)

   _____

   _____

   _____

   _____

5

Setting Goals and Objectives

This may seem like a lot of work, but it clarifies what you do for a living. This is the first step in lesson planning.

Every time I tell a new instructor that I expect goals and objectives written for every class, I get such a look of pain and dismay that it is almost funny. It seems reasonable, they say, for all-day workshops, but do I really expect it for one-hour classes or even half-hour sessions? I do, and it does not take much time or a lot of explanation to convince them why it makes sense.

Think about this. What are you going to teach? How do you know what to include in each class if you don't know what you want the learner to know at the end of your class?

What do you want the learner to know at the end of your class or discussion? That's the goal. A goal is a broad statement of what you want to accomplish. That's it! Just that! It is short, clear, and concise. It doesn't say how you are going to do it, who is going to teach, when it will be done, and how it will be accomplished.

I remember when I realized that goal setting was one of the most important tools an educator had and that it should be done for every class. I was taking a class on writing instructional objectives, and there was a moment in the process that the light went on—this really was important, and I could do it effectively. There is a tiny book titled *Preparing Instructional Objectives*[9] that is part of a classic series for teachers, and I highly recommend it for beginning health care educators. Like its subject matter, it is simple, clear, concise, and a great beginning.

I write goals and objectives for cleaning my living room. It is very clear. The goal: I will have a clean living room. That's it! "I will have a clean living room" is a broad statement of what I want to accomplish. It doesn't define clean. It does not say who is going to clean it. It doesn't say when it will be clean, and it certainly doesn't say how long it will stay clean.

Let's take that to a diabetes education program and look at some sample goals:

- The patient will be able to self-administer insulin.
- The patient will be able to test his blood sugar.
- The patient will be able to count carbohydrates.
- The patient will be able to examine his feet.
- The patient will be able to manage a meal plan.

We can move that out of the diabetes realm, and try the postoperative patient:

- The patient will be able to change his dressing.
- The patient will be able to identify signs and symptoms of infection.
- The patient will be able to ... ?

You may be saying, "Wait a minute—those are all things the patient has to do." Sound familiar? If you did not read Chapter 4

[9] Mager RF: *Preparing Instructional Objectives*. See References.

on the Do-Know-Deficit, go look at it. On the other hand, you will notice there is a word I never used: know. The objective that comes to me stating that the patient or learner will *know* something goes right into the trash. I get thousands of brochures each year for workshops and seminars. I immediately look at the goals and objectives. After all, I want to know what I am going to learn if I go to the workshop. If the brochure says that I will know something, I want to know how they will know that I know something. Will I sit and glow in the dark, or will I sit and grin at them after the program? There is another word that makes me ballistic: recognize. How will the instructor know if I recognize? Will I get all excited and jump up and down? I become very discouraged about our learning process when I see something like that written by otherwise excellent instructors.

If the brochure says I will know about Syndrome X, I want to know what I will have to do to prove that I have learned that. Think about it. Will I have to take a test? Write a sworn statement or testify in court? I need to know that up front because if an examination is involved, you will never see me in that class. I'll bet you feel the same way.

Patients have the same right to know what they are expected to learn and what you will expect them to be able to do at the end of the class.

Let's look at some clear goals for a diabetes education program. For the program itself, here are some samples:

The Diabetes Education Department will

1. present two group programs for the diabetes public in 2003
2. facilitate a multidisciplinary team of a nurse CDE, dietitian, pharmacist, physical therapist, social worker, and physician to design and implement the diabetes patient education series
3. provide a 10-hour diabetes education program on type 2 diabetes
4. develop a 10-hour diabetes education program meeting all the criteria for ADA Recognition

5. implement a diabetes education series utilizing adult education methodology

Take a look at these goals. They tell me what I have to do but give me all the freedom I need to be as creative as I want to. If I presented this to my boss, it would give her an idea of what we would wind up with and the next question would be, how am I going to get there? That requires objectives. We'll get to that below.

Let's look at some goals for actual classes. Here are some examples from my classes:

- meal planning: to provide nutrition education for a patient with diabetes and his or her significant others
- medications: to provide information about the medications that control glucose levels in diabetes
- meal planning: to provide practical tools to assist in meal planning
- psychosocial issues: to provide coping techniques for living with diabetes
- self-care: to teach glucose monitoring

Each of these goals tells you what you will have to teach in the class, clearly, simply, and concisely.

Let's look at objectives. An objective is a simple statement that clearly says what the person will be able to do, at the conclusion of the session, to prove that he or she has learned something. Here are some examples of what you will be able to do after reading this chapter.

At the conclusion of this chapter, the learner will be able to

- define a goal
- write two goals for a diabetes education program
- write a goal for any patient education class
- define an objective
- explain the difference between a goal and an objective
- write five objectives for any class

Do you now have a clear idea of what is taught in this chapter? Objectives tell you what content your class must include. I often talk to new instructors, and the minute they are planning a class, they sit down to write content. How can you do that if you do not know what you want the learner to know at the end of the class? Did you just notice the word know? The question is, what do I want the learner to be able to **do** in order to prove he or she **knows** something?

Remember the goal for cleaning my living room? It was, "I will have a clean living room."

Here are the objectives:

- At the conclusion of the cleaning (this tells me by when) by Ethel (this tells me who is going to do it), there will be (final outcomes)
  - no dust on the furniture
  - no dirt on the floor
  - no magazines on the coffee table
  - no shoes under the couch
  - no gum under the mantle

If these things are true, do I have a clean living room? To me it is clean. I also know, or a cleaning woman will know, what I consider needs to be done in order to have a clean living room. You may consider other things need to be done for the room to be clean. Fine. Write them for cleaning your living room; this is good enough for me.

This brings us to the subject of domains. Bloom's taxonomy defines educational objectives at three levels, cognitive, psychomotor, and affective. A taxonomy is defined as a "mechanism used to categorize things according to their relationships to one another."

The cognitive domain relates to knowledge. What does the person know or need to know, and how do you measure what he or she knows?

When you write an objective, ask yourself the question, what does this person have to do to prove that he knows this subject?

At this point, you use an active verb. He has to explain, describe, identify, list, etc. If the objective states that he will explain the difference between type 1 and type 2 diabetes, then you need to explain the difference in your class. If the objective states that he will list the signs and symptoms of type 2 diabetes, then that is the content and it must be delivered in the format of a list. These are the easiest objectives to write, and I find very few instructors who have difficulty conceptualizing knowledge in this framework.

When I first started writing objectives, I found myself using the same active verbs to the point that it became boring. I found a list of cognitive verbs in an article and posted it over my desk to give me alternatives. It might be helpful for you to do the same.

The psychomotor domain relates to a physical skill. If you want to find out whether people can achieve a physical skill, have them show you that they can do it. Such an objective may be: At the conclusion of the class, the learner will be able to return-demonstrate how to use a lancing device to obtain blood for glucose testing.

I would like to caution you. Do not say that the patient will demonstrate. Instructors demonstrate and students redemonstrate or give return demonstrations. An instructor is the only one who can show you how to do something. This does not mean that you cannot use a student to teach something, but it must be under the supervision of a competent teacher or instructor. When you document, you state that you demonstrated and that the learner was able to redemonstrate, for instance, how to self-administer insulin.

I remember taking an exam as a student nurse. I was asked to write all the steps to preparing a bed for a patient returning from the OR. In those days, they were called "ether beds." Figure that out. I wrote the exam and got a great grade, but it occurred to me that if they wanted to know whether I could make the bed, with all the right equipment, they should let me make one and then check it out.

This is very simple and easy to write and accept. These are the physical skills that patients need and are very easy to prove. These are called competency-based skills. The person can or cannot administer insulin. Think about some of the things that you teach patients that are in the psychomotor domain: self-monitoring of blood glucose (SMBG), blood pressure measurement, dressing changes, etc. Please remember that all of these skills have cognitive and affective components attached, but they are initially physical skills. After all, what is the benefit of taking a blood pressure accurately if you do not know what the reading means or how it affects your life?

The affective domain concerns attitudes or feelings. This is the hardest domain to deal with, whether it is writing objectives, measuring them, or teaching. What can you say or ask that will prove how a learner feels about something?

What if you discussed all the complications of diabetes that can occur if patients do not achieve glycemic control? Then you led a group discussion on the importance of glycemic control and the DCCT study? You might have an objective that says: At the conclusion of the session, the participant will be able to discuss how he will control his blood sugar and the ramifications of poor control. This objective shows that the patient has discussed the importance of glycemic control and accepts that there are ramifications and actually talks about his feelings.

You could also use an objective that actually says, Patient verbalized his concern (feelings) about having to live with diabetes for the rest of his life. It works with any type of class. In a prenatal class, you might write an affective objective that says, At the conclusion of the class, the patient will be able to discuss her feelings of being overwhelmed with the preparations for labor and delivery.

When you start to measure the outcomes of your program or evaluate the session, it will be very easy. If you said the person could list the signs and symptoms and he or she can, you have succeeded in meeting your objectives.

These are called behavioral objectives. Some sources call them terminal behavioral objectives and require that you write interim objectives that explain what the learner will be doing on the way to reaching the terminal or final objective. I think that this is too complicated and unnecessary, but for the sake of the obsessive-compulsive people, I will demonstrate.

If the patient has had a CVA and if partially paralyzed, the goal may be: The patient will be able to go to the bathroom independently.

The objectives will then follow as:

- At the end of one week of physical therapy, the patient will be able to transfer from bed to a standing position, with the assistance of one person.
- At the end of two weeks of physical therapy, the patient will be able to transfer from the bed to a standing position using a walker.
- At the end of four weeks of physical therapy, the patient will be able to walk, with the walker, from the bed to the bathroom, open the bathroom door, enter the bathroom, close the bathroom door, and sit on the toilet. The patient will then complete the toileting and return to the bed.

If the person meets all of the objectives, has he or she met the goal of independent bathroom visits? Yes.

Let's write a goal and three objectives for SMBG. Just to make it interesting, we will write one objective for each of the domains.

- Goal: The person with diabetes will be able to perform SMBG.
- Objectives: At the conclusion of the class, the participant will be able to
  - list the times and reasons for SMBG (cognitive)
  - return-demonstrate how to test blood on his own meter (psychomotor)
  - explain how SMBG gives him control to make decisions about how he manages his diabetes (affective)

The active verbs are list, return-demonstrate, and explain. The content of the class is now defined. You need to list the times and reasons for SMBG, demonstrate the procedure, have the patient return the demonstration, and explain how SMBG gives him control. The evaluation process is then concise. Can the patient meet the objectives? Great!

Here is another example outside of the diabetes realm. A person with a new colostomy has to change her appliance when she goes home.

- Goal: The patient will be able to change her colostomy bag.
- Objectives: At the conclusion of the session, the patient will be able to
  - remove the used colostomy bag and dispose of it in a plastic bag without spilling the contents
  - cleanse the skin around the stoma of fecal matter, using a nonabrasive cloth or tissue
  - wash the area around the stoma using a mild soap and water solution, rinse, and dry without scratching the area
  - demonstrate the correct technique and materials necessary to prepare the skin for the bag application
  - return demonstrate how to apply a clean, correctly sized colostomy bag, using the technique previously demonstrated by the stoma therapist
  - discuss when to change her colostomy bag
  - discuss the importance of privacy and self-respect when changing the bag
  - list some products that can be used to control odor and avoid embarrassment

Document, and go home.

6

How to Motivate People to Learn

Here is my advice on how to get people turned on to you and how to get them motivated to take care of themselves.

I used to believe, when I was first an educator, that if the learner didn't learn, then the teacher didn't teach. I took all the guilt and responsibility and piled it up and lived with it. If you don't know where I'm going with this concept, look at the educators around you. A lot of them still believe that garbage and carry it like a weight on their shoulders.

They believe that if their patient didn't learn, then they didn't teach correctly and should be held responsible. I was going to educate everybody in the world and make sure each person with diabetes received all the information they needed whether they wanted it or not. I finally reduced that to the East Coast of the United States. Now, I'm doing work in all parts of the world, and the difference is that I am not responsible to everybody anymore. Along the road, the patient and I became partners, and we are in this together. Nobody died and left me in charge.

Am I saying that I can't do this without you? Every person I teach, every person who has a health care background, every one of us who comes in contact with people who need education and information needs you. You are so valuable. Now I'm going to try to motivate these people.

Find Out Who You're Teaching

- What's important to them?
- What do they care about?
- What are the barriers?
- How do you tear down the barriers?
- How do you turn them on?

How do you motivate people? First, you have to find out who they are. You have to get to them where they live and deep inside where they exist. You are not talking to a glass of water or a pitcher. You are talking to a human being who has come to you for a life-long learning experience. Some of them are very good at dealing with this major change in their lives, and some are terribly bad. Many of them are angry and in denial. They want no part of the diabetes business and resent anyone who is not willing to tell them that all of this is one great mistake and will be gone very quickly.

A lot of you who work in the community have people who come and bring their baggage with them. I'm not just talking about the shopping cart with everything they've ever owned, but all the bad experiences they've had in their life. The saddest thing I can tell you is that if you get involved with people with diabetes, it is a fact that they're going to bring the trash that some of the health care people have loaded on them in terms of bad care. Many of them have been out there in the world, the real world, and they have been lied to by health care professionals. "You can have chicken but don't eat the candy bar." They have been given misinformation or no information during important events in their lives. They may no longer trust or believe us. They may have gone into the hospital and then home with a brand new baby without anyone telling them how to adequately care for a newborn. There may have been a crisis or even a health care tragedy. How many of you have had a bad experience with health care? And supposedly, we know how to work the system. So, when you want to educate people, you have to get rid of all that garbage. You need to say to them, "I'm here to help you," but they've heard that before; and you might tell them, "I'm here to do this for you," and they've heard that before. We sometimes tell patients that "if you do what I tell you, you'll be all right," and they've heard that statement before as well. We're dealing with all the trash that stays around, all of it.

When I see a patient for an initial interview, the first thing I ask is, "How do you feel about this? You've just been told you're diabetic, you have diabetes. How do you feel about this?" If the first health care person they meet says to them, "You can't do this, or this, or this, or this, and you have to do this for the rest of your life," how do you think they are going to respond? People have said to them, "I'm gonna tell you what you have to do," instead of asking them, "What is important to you? What do you want? How do you feel about all the things that are happening to you at this time?"

You were just told you have diabetes. "I don't want to be a diabetic. Right?" And I say to them, "All right. I don't want to be short. Okay? I'm not getting taller, and your diabetes is not going away. I can teach you how to manage it. I can teach you how to deal with it. It's much better now then it was 20 years ago. We have new medications and treatments, we have new equipment, we have funding now, and we have a lot of other things. You're going to spend the rest of your life dealing with diabetes. It's not going away. It doesn't take a holiday. It doesn't take a day off. You can't say one day I'm not taking my insulin shots today because I need a vacation from diabetes."

I have hypertension. Is that stupid? I have high blood pressure. You know, my parents gave it to me. It has nothing to do with my lifestyle. (Well, maybe it does!) I take all these medications on a regular basis. I have these medications in this medication container, and I tell people that I have a choice. When I teach patients,

I take out my pillbox and show it to them. It has become a great teaching tool. I say to my patients, "You don't want to be a diabetic. Okay. I don't want to have hypertension either. Let me see. This is my choice: take my pills or have a heart attack or a stroke. Now, which do I want? Heart attack, stroke, or pills? I'll take my pills." You don't see me in a gym class. I have to lose weight, 20 pounds, because I can't stand it when I am too heavy. I know the reasons why I should lose 20 pounds. But the important issue is, what motivates me? I will soon be living in a bathing suit. I hate bathing suits. But what really motivates me? Motivating me to keep my blood pressure under control may not be the issue because my blood pressure's under control; it's perfect. I take my pills. I watch what I eat. In the Florida Keys, where I live all winter, I dance three nights a week and I swim every day. When I get home to New York in the spring, I sit, so I gain weight. My blood pressure remains the same (good medication). What motivates me everyday is that I have to get back into a bathing suit next month. And there's a whole bunch of fishermen on the dock with me. That motivates me.

You need to find out what's important to the patient. You know them a lot better then I do because I see them in an acute care setting when they have just be diagnosed or after a crisis. You may have known many of them for years and know their families and occupations. You might meet them in church or at the Grange meeting, town functions, and school activities. You may already know what turns them on, or you need to seek that knowledge and use it to assist the patient in making decisions. Think about what is important to you. I give patients a choice. I say, "You can be a diabetic, or you can be a person who happens to have diabetes." That's so important. How do you identify yourself as a person? Does your diabetes define you, or are you a human being who happens to have, along with many other qualities, a chronic disease? People with diabetes tell everybody they meet that they're a diabetic. Is that true for you? Visualize this. You're at a party, and you are offered a piece of cake. "No, I can't have any. I'm a diabetic," you respond. I personally have high blood pressure, but I

How Does the Patient See Life with Diabetes?

- Are you a diabetic, or a person who happens to have diabetes?
- What are you willing to do to survive?
  - Follow a meal plan?
  - Exercise?
  - Take medications?
  - Monitor blood sugar?
- What pushes your buttons?
  - What is important to you?
  - What would you go to war for?
  - What is not important?
  - How can we get your significant other involved?

don't tell everybody in the world that I'm a hypertensive. If I go to a party and am offered potato chips, I don't tell my hostess that I cannot eat that because I have hypertension. I have been waiting for years for someone to be offered a chair and hear them respond that they cannot sit down because they are a hemorrhoidic! When you discuss this with patients, please give them a choice. You can be a diabetic, or you can be a person who has diabetes.

Once you identify which choice they make, you can go on. Find out who they are and what is important to them. What do they care about? I had a young man in my class many years ago who was in his early 30s and very discouraged about having diabetes. He said that it was too hard to remember to take his medications and eating right was a burden when he was out in the world, trying to make a living. He was angry and thinking about giving up all the routine and regulations I was suggesting. We started talking about his life and where he wanted to be in 20 years. We discussed what it would take to keep him going and healthy and on a path for a long, healthy, successful life. I knew he was crazy about his 6-year-old daughter as he would often bring in pictures of her for me to see and admire. She was a beautiful little girl with golden hair and big blue eyes. We talked about the future and visualized her wedding day, in about 20 years. I asked him how she would feel, if on this most important day of her life, her daddy were not there to share it with her, because he had felt it was too hard an effort to take care of himself. It was difficult to discuss that issue but important enough to use her future, and his love for her, to motivate him to get through this difficult period of adjustment.

What is important to your patients? What would encourage or motivate them to improve their health and lifestyle? Sometimes you need to ask them. I had a patient in a long-term care facility who really enjoyed knitting and crocheting for her grandchildren. It was a great pleasure in her life, and she spent hours making things and delighted in giving the gifts she created. She was having some difficulty with her vision, and we realized that the peaks and valleys in her blood sugar levels affected her sight. I discussed it with her and her physician, and we made some adjustments in her medication and her meal plan that resulted in better control, and ultimately less vision problems. Her family then came looking for me. They had brought "Mama" all kinds of treats, and she had informed them that she couldn't eat them any longer, and they were furious. What right had I to punish this poor old lady and deny her all the pleasures of life? After all, she was in her 80s, and who cared if she ate fried chicken and her favorite berry pies? I decided that we needed a meeting with the patient and her family. With everyone present, we discussed what the patient wanted. She explained to her daughter that she really had difficulty knitting when her vision was blurring, and it really wasn't a problem to eat a little less and make better choices when filling out her menu with the dietitian. It was more important to make sweaters than eat pie. Let the person who lives the life make the life decisions.

What are the barriers to better self-care? I remember telling people that they could not work the night shift and manage their diabetes. We have come a long way. We know that patients who believe they can succeed have a better chance of succeeding. Self-efficacy,[10] or confidence, affects self-care behavior. If patients have

---

[10] Rubin RR, Peyrot M, Saudek CD: The effect of a diabetes education program incorporating coping skills training on emotional well-being and diabetes self efficacy. See References.

no confidence in their ability to manage their diabetes or deal with the constraints involved, then they will have difficulty adjusting or adhering to the care necessary. Find out what upsets them most, and deal with it before it becomes a serious problem. If the person has a family member with diabetes who has had serious complications, that colors her feelings about her ability to survive the condition without the same ramifications and problems. It is helpful to explain the advances that have been made in diabetes care and the treatment modalities that are available now but were not in the past. I show all patients the DCCT[11] and UKPDS[12] results and show them how we have evidence that glycemic control can make a statistically significant difference. Most of my patients have been very impressed by these statistics and encouraged that they actually can make a difference in their own outcomes.

Ginger's Tenets of Teaching

- Look for the teachable moment—They are so special!
- Teaching can be done anytime
  - Answer a question
  - Ask a question
  - Make it part of every activity
  - Make it fun
- You can teach only once you have motivated people to want to learn

You can tear down the barriers only if you identify them and help patients deal with them as problems or deterrents to their success. You can turn patients on if you don't turn them off with demands that they cannot accept or live with.

You cannot do any teaching until you motivate people to want to learn. If you can convince them that learning what you have to offer will make a difference in the quality of their lives, you have a

[11] DCCT Study. See References.
[12] UKPDS Study. See References.

chance. If they think that you are teaching them as part of a group or just because it is your job, you haven't a prayer.

I learn all the time. I have been teaching patients this for a long time and I still cannot stress it enough. Remember: give them a choice. Who are you? A person with diabetes, or a diabetic? Three months ago, one of the medical directors from a pharmaceutical company gave a workshop, and he said, "Ginger, you know I've heard you say that before, and I take exception with you." I said, "What do you mean?" He said, "I'm not a person with diabetes, I am a diabetic. And that's who I am. I spend more of my life taking care of my diabetes then my medical practice. I spend more of my life being a diabetic than being a father. I spend more of my life taking care of my diabetes and being a diabetic than being a husband. I'm a diabetic. And I don't know if I like hearing you give me that choice." I said, "Well, I'm going to give you that choice, and you can decide." I have been thinking about that conversation and have come to this conclusion. I wish he would reconsider. Someday when he dies, and I hope he is at least 120 when that occurs, what will he want said at his graveside? Would he prefer people say he was a wonderful husband and father? A great scientist and doctor? Or a great diabetic? I will have to ask him the next time I see him. You think about it as well.

7

Evaluation Methodology

*What do we evaluate, you ask? Everything—
your education program, courses, classes,
and department.*

Evaluation is a process or a series of processes that makes us look at what we do and who we are. It is difficult to take the time to build it into your education program, but it validates your practice, and that makes it essential.

Many accrediting agencies are involved in health care, and each of them has specific criteria that must be met in order for you to be considered a legitimate entity. In general, to be reimbursed for your services requires that you define outcomes that can be measured and set up a system of self-evaluation. This sounds quite complex and time-consuming, but it makes sense if you look at it logically and put it in a nonthreatening conceptual framework.

Let's start with your course. Are you teaching the same components year after year? Is every Monday the same class as the last Monday? Do all of these parts need to be

EVALUATION METHODOLOGY 51

taught, or are they outdated? Many of us design a course and then live with it for the rest of our careers. Just because it was good, or even wonderful, when you developed it doesn't mean it should not be upgraded or changed on a regular basis.

Please remember that the world of health care is rapidly changing and the technology of our field is partially responsible for driving the curriculum of your program. In the early 1970s, there was no reimbursement for diabetes education or supplies so there was no need to discuss it in your class or program. In the 1990s, we changed all that, and it should absolutely be a part of your classes. How do patients get reimbursement, and what are they entitled to under Medicare, Medicaid, or private insurance? This is as relevant to your patients as why they should check their blood sugar or get an A1C test every three months.

Look at your program objectively. It does not reflect on you if the components look dated or stale unless you then decide not to update or change the program because it is too much effort or beyond your scope of practice.

Before making any changes in your program, you should have a clear understanding of what the current scope and standards of practice are in your area of interest and training. If you are a nurse in the field of diabetes, you can obtain the Scope and Standards for Diabetes Nursing from the American Association of Diabetes Educators (AADE).[13] You can obtain the Scope and Standards of Diabetes Education from the same source. The American Diabetes Association publishes their *Clinical Practice Recommendations* as a supplement to their journal *Diabetes Care* each January. You are responsible for becoming knowledgeable about diabetes practice if you intend to be a diabetes educator.

If oncology or cardiology is your field, contact the American Heart Association, American Lung Association, or the Oncology Nurses Society for up-to-date information and references.

---

[13] American Nurses Association, American Association of Diabetes Educators: *Scope and Standards of Diabetes Nursing*, Washington, DC, American Nurses Association, 1998.

When evaluating your program, consider the requirements of accrediting agencies. Your education program must achieve Recognition to receive reimbursement from Medicare for services provided by your program. If you plan to achieve Recognition for your education program from the American Diabetes Association, you can obtain the criteria by contacting the association or going online (see References; it is an online application). You can also achieve Recognition from the Indian Health Services if you function under that department. They are currently the only two accreditation entities for Medicare reimbursement.

Even if Recognition is not your goal, following the criteria in the National Standards for Diabetes Self-Management Education will help you develop an excellent education program.[14] Why would you want to develop a program without investigating the existing guidelines or standards? Don't reinvent the wheel. If you choose not to follow these criteria, consider your reasoning. Do you lack community or collegial support, or are you satisfied with developing a mediocre education program?

When evaluating your program, ask what you would want to know about the program. Is it current and valid? Does it still make sense? Are there parts of the course that are no longer relevant to the audience? Are there new technologies to add, e.g., pump therapy or computer software for diabetes management?

You do not have to do this evaluation alone. There are many references available to help you look into state-of-the-art programs and models of excellent curricula. In 1997, the Canadian Diabetes Association developed an entire program, including all components, and published it as a manual.[15] I cite this resource because it is a wonderful program and also to encourage you to broaden your scope. I have had wonderful experiences meeting with edu-

[14] American Diabetes Association: National Standards for Diabetes Self-Management Education. See References.

[15] Canadian Diabetes Association Diabetes Education Program: *Patient Education Resource Kit*. Toronto, Ontario, Canada, Canadian Diabetes Association, 1997.

cators from around the world and learning about their programs and processes. We Americans tend to believe that we are the leaders in education around the world, but there are magnificent programs in many other countries.

It is very helpful to allow your advisory board the opportunity to evaluate your program periodically. Please see Chapter 10, Developing an Education Program, for information on your advisory board.

I highly recommend the use of focus groups composed of patients to help you evaluate your course and classes. People who have participated in your program are in a wonderful position to look back at their experience and give you advice. Even if they provided you with written evaluations at the end of your course, six months or a year later, they will be much more objective and capable of telling you how the program met, or did not meet, their needs and the impact it has had on their lives.

Some educators are terrified to put themselves through the evaluation process. Our egos tend to be fragile little things, and we hate to have missed the boat or disappointed anyone. What if the evaluations are not perfect, and you have to submit them to your boss? It is threatening if the security of your job is at stake.

Most evaluations done at the end of a class or course are just popularity contests. We want to know whether people like us and enjoyed the course. Be honest with yourself. We all want people to like, and maybe love, us. I really care about my patients, and they know that. They hesitate to tell me anything negative because they certainly don't want to hurt my feelings. After all, I work hard, and they know I mean well. Sound familiar?

Asking them to submit something anonymously six months later may get you a more objective evaluation. What if you sent them a form and a stamped, self-addressed envelope to mail to you six months after the program? What if another educator called and spoke to them about the program? Would the evaluation be more accurate if you had prepped them to expect it, had told them that you were looking for the truth, and explained that you need their help keeping your class as up-to-date and as good as you wanted it to be? Could you assure them that your job would not be in danger if they said anything unfavorable about you, the other instructors, or the program?

What value does your program have for the patient? This is your opportunity to measure the outcomes. The ADA Education Recognition Program requires that you set up a system of outcomes measurements to assure that your program is making a difference in the lives of the patients who participate.

Requirement 10 of the National Standards for Diabetes Self-Management Education (DSME) Programs states that, "The DSME entity will use a continuous quality improvement process to evaluate the effectiveness of the education experience provided and determine opportunities for improvement."

What does that mean? You could choose any number of clinical indicators to evaluate the effectiveness of the program. For example, you could say that the patient's A1C will drop from 11% to 9% within six months after he or she participated in your program. Weight changes, BMI, cholesterol levels, BP—these are all acceptable parameters to monitor and a valuable way to see whether you make a difference in a patient's health care status. CMS, the Centers for Medicare and Medicaid Services (formerly the Health Care Finance Administration), requires that you document outcomes for your patients to receive reimbursement under Medicare.

The required outcomes have you collecting data on the following:

- education goals
- duration of diabetes
- medications
- height and weight
- lab work on lipids
- blood pressure
- eye exam and date
- self-monitoring of blood glucose
- assessment on educational needs
- evaluation of program and patient goals
- evaluation methodology
- follow-up plans for 6 months and 1 year
- continued follow-up with primary care provider

You will notice that most of these are clinical indicators that will tell you whether your patient's health status is improving, remaining the same, or declining. This is important information.

In diabetes care, there are other things we want to know. The AADE has developed a program called the National Diabetes Education Outcomes System (NDEOS). It measures behavioral changes, which gives you an opportunity to look at the changes a patient may make in his or her life because he or she attended your program. Review the program on the AADE web site (www.aadenet.org); it may give you new insight on the importance of doing a quality improvement evaluation program.

The NDEOS measures patients' behaviors and identifies their priorities for change. The seven diabetes education outcomes areas identified are

- physical activity
- food choices
- medication administration
- monitoring of blood glucose
- problem solving for blood glucose, high, low, sick days
- risk-reduction activities
- psychosocial adaptation (living with diabetes)

Remember, no matter what kind of patient education program you run, there should be some kind of measurement system in place so you can justify the program as beneficial to the patients or community you serve. Perhaps you are doing asthma education. The clinical indicator you build into the program might be that the person will not have to use a rescue inhaler more that three times per week. For a cardiac rehabilitation program, you might identify the indicator that the patient will increase his or her physical activity to walking one mile at least three times per week.

It is not that difficult to prove that what you do for a living is important and makes an impact on people's lives.

How do you evaluate your classes? In Chapter 8, Creative Teaching Techniques, I cover this thoroughly. I encourage you to set up a formal evaluation mechanism and schedule the evaluations on a regular basis.

There are all kinds of resources available to assist you. In acute care settings and hospitals, there are quality improvement managers whose main function is to set up systems throughout the facility to provide quality data for accrediting bodies. These colleagues would be the logical candidates to assist you in developing the process for your outpatient clinic or office. It is in their best interest to invest in improving the quality of care for their patients by collaborating with other health care facilities or entities in the community. It will also give them the opportunity to benchmark programs in larger areas and collect data that would be useful in public health arenas.

Talk to the Public Health Department in your area and ask them to lend you an intern from their department to help you develop your system. These are usually people in a master's program in public health or health care administration, and while they can be of great use to you, they get the knowledge and experience you can share with them from the real world.

It can be very disconcerting when an administrator or surveyor approaches you and asks how you know that your program is of value or worth the money the facility is spending to maintain your department. It feels great when you can say, "Let me show you the data we have collected and the money we are saving the health care system by cutting hospital readmissions for patients post-op cardiac surgery." Or "Look at the number of patients who are no longer being admitted every year for diabetes complications." Then it sounds like you know what you're doing!

8

Creative Teaching Techniques

Here I get to do what I love to do best, teaching health care providers to teach creatively. We are here to have fun!

Why should you use different techniques? If you bore people, they won't learn. Look at the people in your classes. Look at the body language. I recommend a book that was written years ago, titled *Body Language*.[16] It talks about how people demonstrate their feelings with their body. Are people in your classes bored? Does the time drag? Does anyone fall asleep? To me, being boring should be a capital crime.

If you do the same thing the same way all the time, you will burn out and drive yourself out of the business. You need to find ways to keep yourself motivated. Be creative and share with all your friends and colleagues. We'll discuss that further below. If you are bored, it will come across to your patients. Remember, you may be teaching that foot care class for the hundredth time, but it's the

---

[16] Fast J: *Body Language*. See References.

Keep Yourself Motivated

- Use different teaching techniques, or
  - You'll bore the patient
  - You'll bore yourself
  - You won't want to continue
- You need to have fun
  - We wear too many hats to start from scratch

- Look for alternative teaching methods
  - How do people learn?
  - How do you learn?
  - What do you want them to learn?
  - What do you have available?
  - Who can teach for you?
  - Who can you learn from?

---

patient's first time to hear what you have to say, and he needs to know this important material. You cannot walk in and think, "Not this class again." If you are sick of a class, you will never do it well; find other ways, or someone else, to teach it.

You need to enjoy your classes and have some fun. We work too hard not to have fun at what we do. If you are like 90% of the educators I know, you work late and you are there for everyone. Many of us wear several hats. You may be a diabetes, cardiac, or surgical instructor. Perhaps you cover for supervisors or do staff development. Can you do everything you do, be all things to all people, and survive to return another day? Certainly. Many of us do this for years, and love it, but in order to do it, you must enjoy it and have fun.

Don't start from scratch. There is so much information, you have no need to start from the beginning. It has taken us 30 years to get to this stage, and just because you may be new to the business doesn't mean you have to pay all the dues that we have had to pay in the past. Talk to the experienced people who have had to learn, or even invent, the materials and techniques we use in this enlightened era.

Look for alternative teaching methods. How do people learn? How do you learn? We talked about that in Chapter 3, The Adult Learner. Read it again if you need to.

When you are planning your classes, remember how people learn. If you are a visual learner, and people show you something once, you will remember it. I can close my eyes and visualize an entire class that I attended years ago. Every so often, I'll need help on a PowerPoint project, so I call my son who teaches this for a living. He will ask, "Did you look in the manual?" Do I have time to look in the manual? He sent manuals to me, and they are gathering dust at the corner of my desk. If I had time to do that, I could be writing more chapters of this book!

That is not how I learn. Ask your patients how they learn. For example, I hand people a box with a meter. Everything is in there, instructions, long and short versions, a videotape, etc. Do they open the box and read everything and learn? No. They say, "Show me." At some point in their lives, they decided that the way they learn best is to have someone show them how to do something, so I have to show them. They are entitled to learn the way they learn best. Did you learn to drive a car by reading a book?

Years ago, I got a call from a nurse on a patient unit when I was director of staff development. She said that a new midstream urine kit had appeared on the floor and no one knew how to use it— would I come up and show them? I had never seen the kit, so I got one from central supply and read the box and enclosed instructions in the elevator on my way to the unit. It didn't seem like a big deal to me; the instructions were simple, clear, and concise. It occurred to me that it was amazing: although both of us were RNs, we approached this learning situation differently. I read the box and went up to teach the procedure to another RN. But, why didn't she just read the box and do the procedure? I don't think I am so much smarter; she must have seen that as my job. She obviously felt that she would learn it easier and faster if I went upstairs and showed her how to do it, so I earned my paycheck.

When I first taught a "diabetic diet," what we now call a meal plan, I would bring people together in the hospital lounge to share lunch. They would look at each other's meal and compare what they were eating. We used real food because I could not afford to buy food models. The patients would look at each other's trays and become jealous. A patient would ask, "Why does he have two pieces of bread, when I have only one?" "He exercises or he does-n't have to lose weight," I would answer. "If I exercise or lose some weight, can I have two?" the patient would respond. "Sure. His blood sugar doesn't go up when he eats one slice of bread," I would say. "Does mine?" he would ask. "Check your blood with your meter," I would say. Look what I have accomplished: Perhaps he will be motivated to exercise or test his own blood with a meter.

Who can they learn from? Who can teach them best?

It is now time to evaluate our courses, our classes, and . . . take a deep breath . . . our teaching techniques.

Our Courses

How many sessions are they? Are they the same sessions you have always taught? Are they three hours long? How long do you make the patients sit there? Are there games and activities? Do you change your techniques every few minutes? Do you find ways to keep people awake, alert, and interested? I give prizes in my courses. We play games and do activities and people win prizes. They love the little things that I buy at the dollar store. Often I ask the industry representatives for little giveaways to use, and it saves me money and shopping time.

I was tired of people coming late to class, so I stood at the door and handed prizes to the first three people in class. I knew it was working when people were racing down the hall to win a post-a-note pad! Some classes are in the evening, and people come after work. I blow whistles, play games, and do activities.

Evaluation Time

Our courses
- How many sessions?
- What do we teach now?
- Have you done a Do-Know-Deficit lately?

Our classes
- How long?
- Who teaches them?
- What is taught?
  - Needs to know
  - Wants to know
  - Nice to know

People want us to validate our classes. It has been suggested that we give our patients tests to measure outcomes. Adults don't like tests! You tell me that I have to take a test, and I am gone. How then do I know if they have learned? Play Jeopardy. If they get the questions right and win money (cheap prizes) with correct information, I know what they know. If they answer incorrectly, we go over the correct information. It is fun, they learn, and they come back to class. Sometimes they keep coming, and I have to remind them that enough is enough. Do you have people who have become groupies? I finally had to tell one of my favorite patients that she really did not have to come anymore and was probably qualified to teach most of my classes.

Here is a suggestion. Make a simple board with "pockets" similar to those libraries use in the back of their books to hold due-date cards. Then make up answers to content questions and put them in the pockets. Each person gets a whistle, bell, or horn, and if someone answers a question correctly, he accumulates fake money and uses the money to get prizes. Everybody gets prizes anyway. If there are too many people, form competing teams. Adults love to compete. New Yorkers get crazy when they lose, so be careful. No one is a "loser."

If students have learned the topic quickly, save the time for another subject. Have them show you what they can do, and validate that they did it correctly. If they need to unlearn and relearn, then you will have the extra time because you saved it from an earlier experience.

Don't assume that your course has to stay the same because it always was this way and it is successful. The world, and people, change. If you evaluate, and it is still valid and wonderful, fine—don't change just for the sake of changing.

Our Classes

How do you evaluate your class? How long is your class? Is it too long for people who have worked a whole day? If you do evening classes, would the group rather come five weeks for two hours at

Creative Teaching Techniques Idea List

- Discover what materials and resources are available
- Watch and talk to the professional educators
- Do you need to teach every class yourself? Ask colleagues to guest teach
- Try finding 5 different ways to teach the same thing
- Try exercises, games, and ice breakers
- Ask the patients how they want to learn!
- Create a Patient Education Team
- Can your course or class be a Quality Improvement Project?
- Use materials from other professionals
- Get funding for materials, guest speakers
- Find out what your professional associations have to offer
- Find out what local colleges/universities have to offer
- Ask for donations of materials

a time than three weeks for three hours? Ask them what they want at the first meeting. Does it have to be the same every time? Do you have alternatives, and do you give the students the choice of which one is more convenient for their lifestyle?

Are you playing games and getting people up and doing something? Do you put on slides or movies and shut off the lights? Never let people sit in a dark room—they go to sleep. Use an audiovisual that allows light in the room so you can watch people's faces. This will give you an indication of how they are doing.

Who teaches the class? Are you alone, or do you find colleagues to help? If you need a dietitian and do not have one in your program, borrow someone from the dietary or food service department, the local WIC program, public health, or a local nursing home or hospital. You will find someone who loves to teach people, and if he is new at teaching but knows his stuff when it comes to your topic, teach him how to teach. For most of my career, I have identified a very skilled, competent nurse in the hospital and recruited him or her for staff development. Then I would teach him how to teach. You can find a social worker, physical therapist, pharmacist, or even a physician who would love to be in your program. Ask!

When you team teach, you add energy to the room. Each person who gets up is ready, willing, and excited about doing his or her part. I always stick around to help them (they call it butting in) should they need assistance with their section.

We are lucky to have colleagues in each profession who can bring their expertise to the program. Include them, and you will see a change in the dynamics of your program. Remember the foot care class that I really don't love to teach? Well, who loves feet? Podiatrists. Get a podiatrist to teach it for you. They will enjoy it and might even get referrals for patients out of the deal. Why not? It's good for your patients to see a podiatrist, and most visits are covered by insurance. I beg you, however, never to invite people to lecture until you have seen them teach. Just because they are brilliant doesn't mean they know how to teach or can come across to an audience. You may have to prepare their materials and/or teach them how to teach. But it's better than the alternative: If they stand up and read their notes, it will be deadly.

Our Teaching Techniques

What materials are available? We are very fortunate that the pharmaceutical companies provide all kinds of materials for us to use with our patients. Each company has handouts and even games that it is willing to give us free of charge. You don't have to develop a manual anymore because there is an amazing amount of books available that were developed by wonderful, competent people who can save you months of work and time. Don't reinvent the wheel. Look at the resources I have provided for you in the References.

Share with your colleagues. Be aware, however, that we tend to have health care tunnel vision, looking only to our own fields for information and materials. This is a natural phenomenon as we all seek out our comfort zone. Look at the people sitting together in any hospital or university cafeteria: the dietitians are together, the nurses gather in one corner, and the physicians usually have their own dining room. We talk about our own fields, business, or concerns. We need to move outside of that space and talk and learn from new people.

Check out the universities that have teaching colleges. They have wonderful resources available in their bookstores. A fun course at a college for primary or secondary schoolteachers could inspire and motivate you. There are wonderful stores made for elementary schoolteachers in which I love to browse. It's very motivating. I always buy games and activities there and convert them for my adult patients. It is amazing to me that it usually takes very little conversion.

I found a wonderful series of books called *Games Trainers Play*.[17] The materials can be used for all kinds of classes. The resources can be endless and just have to be found. There are all kinds of materials available from the Federal Government, and they are free of charge to anyone. The National Diabetes Education Program has developed hundreds of materials that you can obtain free and use for your patients. Look at the web sites of the nonprofit organizations for what they offer about their subjects. The American Dietetic Association and the Lung Association are great places to start. If you are a surgical nurse, look to your association. The Oncology Nurses Society has materials for professionals that have been tested and validated by the professionals in their field.

If your foot care class needs more energy, go to the local podiatry college and see what they have available. I spoke to a podiatrist who donated a large plastic foot for my class that raised the enthusiasm and interest of the class.

If you work in a hospital, when another service or department holds seminars or workshops, stop by and see what they are doing. Collect the handouts and talk to the pharmaceutical representative, whom you may not know. He or she may have materials that are relevant to one of your classes.

Look at your audiovisual techniques. What do you use for class? If you are still using transparencies, maybe it's time for you to look at PowerPoint. Can your slides whiz in and out? What about

[17] Newstrom JW, Scannell EE: *Games Trainers Play*. See References.

videos in the middle of a program, with pictures of the people in the class. Think about Disney World—there is nothing boring there. People love to see photos of themselves screaming on the rides.

I recommend that you give patients a videotape of your class. Find a day when your hair looks great and you don't feel fat. Have someone tape you and duplicate the tape for your patients. You can have the patients bring you blank tapes to save you money. When patients are handed a commercial tape, they may or may not watch it at home. This really kills me; I have made tapes for several companies and can only hope that people watch them. But when they have a tape featuring their teacher, they will show it, and you, to their families and really watch it. If you are uncomfortable taping it yourself, go the community cable station and ask them to help or do it for you. They must perform a certain amount of free work for the community in order to keep their licenses, so they will be glad to help. If you do not have a community cable, try the local college or university audiovisual department or school of communications. This is a wonderful project for an undergraduate or graduate student. You may want to try creating an audiotape that people can play in the car while they are commuting. Many pharmaceutical or health companies have these tapes made already. Give them to your students. CD-ROMs are everywhere, and the companies are glad to give them to you for your use. The slides they develop are done by professionals, and you can copy some of them for your own programs for patients. They are delighted to let you use them.

Here is an often overlooked resource: University students are always looking for projects, and they might be glad to help you develop a game, create a tape, or translate a manual into a language you need for your multicultural population.

How do you teach the same subject five different ways? Take a short course or class that you know well and look at it. Take the time to really be creative and think of five different ways you could teach this class. It will be very difficult the first time and get easier each time you do it. If you get your colleagues, or your teaching group, together and do it like an arts and crafts party, it could be great fun. One day, I finished teaching a fun class for 4,000 people at the American Association of Diabetes Educators annual meeting. They seemed to love it, and I was feeling pretty good about myself. My dear friend Betty Brackenridge came over, congratulated and kissed me, and then offered to help jazz up my slides. You can never be too good to get help from your friends!

Try new teaching techniques. Do "ice breakers" the first class, so the students get to know each other and bond at the beginning. They will discover what they have in common, and you will find out about the human beings you are teaching. Look into games, exercises, and activities. How about dancing the Electric Slide or Bunny Hop in your class on exercise? Here is a fun, cheap ice breaker: Bring a role of toilet paper to class. Give the first person the roll and ask her to take as little or as much paper as she likes and pass the roll on to another person. Wait until everyone has some paper from the roll. Then ask them to separate their paper into the little sheets by tearing them at the perforations. Some people will have only a few sections and some greedy people will have lots. They then have to stand up in turn and tell the group something about themselves. They have to tell one thing for each piece of paper in their pile. Some patients have resorted to the names of each of their kids for each piece. By the end of the exercise, you have a cohesive group of people who know each other and will be a lot more comfortable sharing their concerns about living with diabetes.

What resources and tools are available? Many of our friends and colleagues have developed games—wouldn't it be fun to share all these games? See below!

Dig up some funds. Many local service groups would be glad to sponsor a health education program or the development of a teaching game or tool. You just need to ask. If they don't have money, perhaps they can provide time or materials. Ask the local print shop about donating paper or transparencies. Would a local computer store help you redo your teaching slides in PowerPoint if you buy the program? There is money out there. Go to the Lion's Club and the Rotary. They may not give you a million dollars, but you could probably get $100 to buy some food models.

Can your students help? They have all kinds of skills and abilities. Perhaps your class holds a computer expert who can convert your transparencies into computer files. Perhaps someone will download materials from the Internet for you. Patients love to teach their instructors and give something back to the people who help them so much.

How about your friends? Can your friends do things to help you with your projects? I bet you know very capable people who would be glad to make the games for you. My husband has a workshop and makes many of my games.

Finally, I urge you to take an impartial, honest look at yourself. This is the hardest thing I will ask you to do. Let someone you trust videotape you and look at how you appear to a class. It will really shock you. Do you wipe your nose or scratch something? Are you redundant? Do you look at people when you teach? Do you turn your back on the audience? This may be the most important thing you ever do but the most insightful and difficult. No one likes to appear, or feel, foolish in public. Remember all of the studies showing that people would rather die than do public speaking? You speak in public for a living, so you are a very brave soul. Good for you.

I remember having my husband in one of my early classes. As I walked up and down the aisle, he grabbed my skirt and whispered, "If you say 'okay' one more time, I will kill you." Okay! I no longer use that word.

Please have fun! You work too hard not to have fun when you teach! Good luck finding the joy in teaching.

Now, here's an example of how to find some wonderful tools. I sent the following e-mail to some of my friends and colleagues:

My dear friends, I am working on the final stages of my book and am taking advantage of our friendship to ask a favor. One of the sections of my book, Creative Teaching Techniques, contains games, exercises, or toy ideas that I have used in my classes over the years. I am asking you to send me one of yours, if you would care to share it with me and the world . . . etc.

Here are the results.

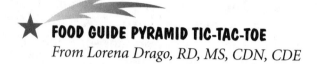

★ **FOOD GUIDE PYRAMID TIC-TAC-TOE**
From Lorena Drago, RD, MS, CDN, CDE

This team game reviews the Food Guide Pyramid, food groups, serving sizes, and healthy eating. You will need a flip chart, markers, prepared questions, tape, and 9 game pieces per team, such as index cards decorated with stickers of orange or apples (from a school or office supply store) to designate the teams. Don't forget the prizes!

On the flip chart, draw a tic-tac-toe grid big enough for the game pieces. Divide the class into two teams; have each choose a team captain. Flip a coin to see which team gets the first question from you. The team has 30 seconds (or some time you designate) to come up with the correct answer, conveyed by the captain. Instead of team captains, players could alternate answering questions. A correct answer means the team fills in a space of their choice on the tic-tac-toe grid with their game piece. If answered incorrectly, the other team gets a chance to answer that question. First team with 3 in a row wins.

Vary your questions in difficulty suitable to the players' knowledge of material; make them true/false or multiple choice. Here are some sample true/false questions.

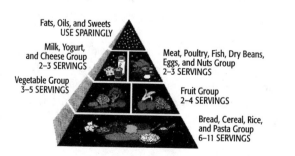

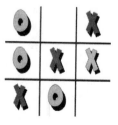

Tic Tac Toe Squares

1. Carrots, green peas, and spinach are examples of protein foods.
2. Peanut butter does not have cholesterol.
3. Wheat bread is a whole grain, and it is high in fiber.
4. Dark green leafy vegetables are good sources of vitamins A and C.
5. Canola and olive oils are saturated fats.
6. Chicken breast without skin is a high-fat meat.
7. We should have at least five servings of fruits and vegetables a day.
8. Oranges and beans are good sources of folic acid.
9. Yellow and orange fruits like apricots, cantaloupes, and peaches are good sources of vitamin A.
10. Potatoes, cantaloupes, and bananas are good sources of potassium.
11. Low-fat foods, such as skim or 1% milk, are good sources of calcium.
12. One cup of corn flakes has more fiber than one cup of oatmeal.
13. Rye and 100% whole-wheat bread have more fiber than white bread.
14. Spinach, kale, and collard greens are good sources of folic acid.
15. A fresh fruit is a better choice than fruit juice.

Answers

1. False	4. True	7. True	10. True	13. True
2. True	5. False	8. True	11. True	14. True
3. False	6. False	9. True	12. False	15. True

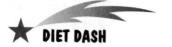

★ **DIET DASH**
From Maggie Forys, MPH, RD, CDE

This is a relay game to play with children at camp. Print large pictures of various foods from available clip art on card stock using an ink-jet printer. Take them to a teacher's supply store and laminate them very inexpensively.

Create a poster with paper bags and write the names of different food groups, carbohydrate, fat, protein, mixed meal, etc., on each of the bags.

Divide the kids into teams. The players are handed a card with a food on it. They have to run to the bags and put the food in the correct bag before they can go back and tag the next member of their team. The first team done with all their cards signals.

The bags are then checked for correct cards, and the team with the most correct wins prizes. There are prizes for the runners-up, so no one is disappointed.

The kids have fun and learn too!

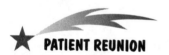

★ **PATIENT REUNION**
From Cindy Merrins, MHS, RD, BC-ADM, CDE

I like to have a reunion for the many patients in our clinic who have fallen out of touch with us. We usually have a Spring Fling and a Fall Festival, with about 40 patients invited to each, based on having about two or three programs in a 6-week period. We look for those patients we need to check on. About 30 will show up. Interwoven in our program and entertainment are several messages: getting flu shots, checking BP, communicating with health care providers, etc. We have had schoolchildren from the community sing and local entertainers at different occasions. Sometimes we play Diabetes Bingo.

Start with a regular bingo set. Instead of the letters B-I-N-G-O, I put different colors across the top of the bingo card. Instead of the numbers in the columns, I put words like fiber, foot care, meters, or carbohydrates. I would call out "yellow fiber," and they could only cover the space with a chip if they could answer the question that I asked about fiber. I give out prizes that I get from the pharmaceutical company representatives. I have also received cash donations from local companies.

Another teaching technique I have used is an icebreaker where I ask people in the group identify who has had diabetes for 6 months, 1 year, 5 years, etc. Finally, when reviewing nutrition with patients in a group (or doing staff training), I put food models in a grab bag and ask someone to reach in and choose one. We then review everything we can say about that apple or salad dressing, such as, "Is this a carb?" It's lots of fun.

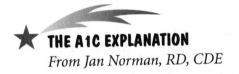

★ THE A1C EXPLANATION
From Jan Norman, RD, CDE

Take an egg-shaped container from a pair of panty hose and attach fuzzy balls from a craft or fabric store using Velcro. Try to get colored balls. The more balls, the higher the A1C. This is a great visual for sticky red blood cells.

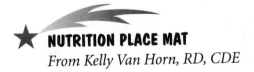

★ NUTRITION PLACE MAT
From Kelly Van Horn, RD, CDE

Go to the web site *www.tabletopnutrition.com* for examples of place mats.

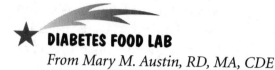

★ DIABETES FOOD LAB
From Mary M. Austin, RD, MA, CDE

In 25 years as an educator of adult learners, I have found that visual, hands-on instruction seems to work best. Retention is greater and learning is more enjoyable when the learner participates in an activity. A particularly popular activity is what I call the "Diabetes Food Lab." The Diabetes Food Lab can be used to meet many different learning objectives.

Objectives

- learn appropriate diabetes food portion sizes as specified in the *Exchange Lists for Meal Planning* or for carbohydrate counting
- identify foods that contain carbohydrate
- identify foods that contain fat
- be able to measure foods accurately
- learn to manage portion control in a restaurant setting

The Diabetes Food Lab can take place in a free-standing diabetes clinic, in the hospital cafeteria, or at a local restaurant. Equipment and food supplies will differ depending on the objective(s) you select and the location you select.

For example, if you want to teach appropriate diabetes food portions in an inpatient or outpatient group setting, you would need the following materials:

- food to be weighed or measured, such as mashed potatoes, rice, popcorn, frozen peas or corn, dry cereals, fruits of various sizes, bagels of various sizes, margarine, salad dressings
- measuring cups and spoons
- postage scale
- paper plates

- paper bowls
- handout listing appropriate food portion sizes (use the *Exchange Lists for Meal Planning* or whatever you currently use for medical nutrition therapy instruction)

Ask each participant to portion out a given amount of the same food on a plate or in a bowl without using measuring utensils. For example, everyone is to portion out what they think 1/2 cup of mashed potatoes looks like. Then ask participants to actually measure and weigh the portion they put on the plate and compare it to the amount listed on their handout. For people who have not weighed or measured foods in the past, they tend to portion out what they typically have had served to them, either at home or in restaurants. This can be very interactive and lively.

Additional Diabetes Food Labs could take place in a hospital cafeteria or restaurant. It is best to conduct the lab in a private area or room in the cafeteria/restaurant and inform the cafeteria/restaurant manager of the class.

Care should be taken to make sure that the participants are not made to feel deficient in their ability to estimate portion sizes, but to have fun while learning a new skill.

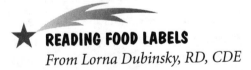

★ READING FOOD LABELS
From Lorna Dubinsky, RD, CDE

This is something I do in my individual counseling when teaching label reading. On a big index card, I put the front of the label with the picture of the food (if enough room) and the Nutrition Facts information. This way, I can compare different foods, and the client can see which would be the better choice for healthy eating and when looking for sodium or saturated fat, etc.

Some foods I use often are cheese (regular, reduced fat, no fat), canned soups and the packaged noodle soups, chips (fried, baked, tortilla), and ice cream (regular, light, no sugar added). It's a lot easier to go through the index cards than a big box of food packages.

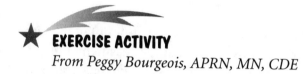

★ EXERCISE ACTIVITY
From Peggy Bourgeois, APRN, MN, CDE

Use videos! A popular exercise video that our patients like is "Walk Away the Pounds with Leslie Sansone." Even our elderly patients like it because they don't like to leave their homes and there are no safety or weather issues. Another popular video is "Angela Lansbury's Positive Moves: A Personal Plan for Fitness and Well-Being at Any Age." This tape was made after she broke her hip and was on a plan to resume exercise and keep weight off. Of course, because he is from New Orleans (my town), anything by Richard Simmons, like "Sweating to the Oldies," is a favorite.

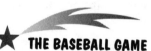

★ THE BASEBALL GAME
From Lois Book, RN, EdD, PhD, CDE

During spring and summer classes, I used a baseball theme in the presentations of group classes. I used the analogy of the three bases for diabetes management: that it takes skill and work to make a hit and get to any of the diabetes control bases. For these classes, I wore a baseball jersey and hat and brought a ball, bat, and gloves to the class and had them represent the nutrition, medication, and monitoring. The theme and nondiabetes props worked very well in keeping it practical and simple. The men in the class especially loved it, and the women could also benefit from the thought process. The RD teacher of the group would say that she did not know much about diabetes and was like them, learning what the game is all about. This allowed talking about the emotions of being unsure, being scared, having a feeling of doubt that you could do it, being scared of what you need to do, having each day different, having to do something with the ball or nutrition, not learning just by reading about it, watching another person do it, needing to learn by doing, talking to others who are doing it, and striking out sometimes but being active. The analogy worked very well.

We also found it very enjoyable for members of the group to be actively involved, such as doing cooking demonstrations. With ingredients on hand, we had one person make something in front of the group that everyone got to taste, like a punch, a pudding, or fruit salad (things that did not need cooking); we shared the expenses involved and had tastings. We actually staged Christmas, New Year's, and Thanksgiving gatherings to show what it takes and how to avoid being tempted by too many sweets and lack of exercise on those days. Having classes in a hospital in the basement next to the dining room and cafeteria really helped.

For staff development in the field of diabetes, I would use costumes while teaching. My most notable was to be the Cat in the Hat. Dressing up to teach in front of a group made it seem more fun when the people arrived in the room and made the participation easier for most because the formalness was broken. Characters by Dr. Seuss and from Charlie Brown and Peanuts were my most enjoyable dress-up themes to use. The concept was to make a warm, accepting learning environment and to stimulate more of the brain to take in the learning while appealing to something familiar.

9

Curriculum Development and Developing Lesson Plans

Now that you have developed your goals and objectives, you are ready to develop your lesson plan.

It is quite simple to put the materials you have already learned into the context of curriculum development. Look at the format below. It is a sample of the kind of tool that will make your work much easier. I am giving you a complete template to duplicate, if you wish, below.

The top of the lesson plan should include the name of the course or class. I like to give it a fun name if possible, so when someone asks me to do a seminar or workshop, I have a catchy title to arouse the interest of the participant. For example, I call my class on motivation of patients "How to Motivate: Or Which Buttons to Push."

Then identify why you are doing this class in the first place, i.e., the goal, which could be insulin self-administration. Then you fill in the columns with the requested information.

The topic is the name of the topic you will be teaching. You have already learned to develop the objectives.

Topic	Objectives	Content	Activities	Time Frame	Instructor
	At the conclusion of the session, the participant will be able to:				
1. Insulin administration	1. Identify his or her insulin(s) correctly from a group of insulins	1. Show all the insulins, and let the patient identify the one(s) to use	1.	1.	1.

They are terminal behavioral objectives, clear and concise, and are always measurable. Number them in the column, and make sure the numbers are continued in each of the additional columns across so that you, or anyone reading the plan, can follow the entire process easily.

Remember that the objective can be any one of the domains, cognitive, psychomotor, or affective. This is your "do." Sound familiar? At the top of the objectives column I write, "At the conclusion of the session, the participant will be able to:". This covers all the objectives, and I do not have to write it before each objective statement. It saves time and makes it clear to the reader.

1. Insulin administration	1. Select the correct insulin from a group of insulins	1. Have the patient select his insulin from a group of insulins. Play the musical insulin game. When the music stops, patients rush to select their correct insulin from the big box of insulins.		

Now that you have identified what the person will be able to do, you are able to fill in the content column. The content is what you will teach people so that they will be able to do what you want them to, in other words, meet the objective. This is the "know" coming to the forefront. Is it beginning to make sense to you?

Be as detailed as you can in this column. Remember that we all get sick, hope to take vacations, and prepare lessons plans for other people. If you think the content is too lengthy for this narrow column, put only the content topics and make a note to see an attached page or PowerPoint presentation. You may also want to attach an article that you used to develop this class or national standards that were your resource. Please remember that if someone else is teaching this class, the audience is still going to ask questions about the content that you prepared, and the instructor has to have the information you had when you developed the content to answer the questions.

I sometimes make myself crazy. I often have to prepare workshops or classes more than six months in advance for a program that may be conducted the following year. When I develop curriculum, I walk around for a few days, or a couple of weeks, thinking about who the audience is and where I want to take the topic. Then I get an idea for a theme or a concept, and I build the entire workshop around that "gimmick." Strange as it may sound, this work may have taken me a month in my head but just three hours on the computer. Anyway, the program then flows, and I send it out. Six months later, I may not remember what I was thinking when I developed it. I look at the program and wonder where I came up with this stuff. If I haven't shirked my job, when I did the lesson plan, I included all the concepts and plans. I just pull it out and am remotivated by the concept I developed the year before. If I did not take the time to do the lesson plan, I am out in deep water without a paddle and may be presenting an entirely different theme than I intended originally. It may be just as good, but I will worry that I missed a very good idea that I had the previous year. Ideas are too exciting to waste.

If you think I am getting out of hand at this point, listen to reason. You are only going to prepare this lesson plan once. You will review and perhaps revise it every six months or so, but the major development will probably be done at this initial stage. Don't scrimp on the work now, or you will find yourself having to go back and add things time and time again. If you are keeping your lesson plans in a loose-leaf binder, you will have the freedom to take out the section as a separate entity when you teach the class or to revise it easily without having to take everything apart.

The next topic is the fun column: activities. How will you teach this content? What games, exercises, didactic, or process will you do to teach the identified content? Here are some clues I have learned from experience. If you are showing a movie, write the name of the movie, who you bought it from, and where to get another copy for a future employer or when it becomes lost. I wish I had some of the books and materials I have lent to people and then forgot who I gave them to so I could not request them back— I probably could fill a library.

If you list a game, make sure the instructions are attached and listed in the column. If the material is shared with someone else or borrowed from another agency or department, make a note where it can be located. I find phone numbers and addresses are helpful. If you choose not to put them in the column, write them on the back of the lesson plan. It will save you lots of time and aggravation.

This is the time to use all your creativity. Use some of the ideas you found in Chapter 8, Creative Teaching Techniques. Sometimes, I list alternatives for the same subject. If I am doing an icebreaker, I might suggest the "toilet paper game" or the "remember the name game," and let the instructor choose which one they feel like playing that day.

The column labeled "Time Frame" is to give you a heads up on how long the class should take you. How long do you think that you have in that class to teach that topic? It varies with the type of group and the situation. Someone will call and ask me to teach a class on patient education. I ask about the target audience first. That will make a major difference in my decisions. I ask what they want the learner to know when he leaves my class. Then I can give them a reasonable estimate of the time I will need to meet the objectives. I am able to project that I can teach that subject for one hour, two hours, five hours, one week, or, as in the case of writing this book, 20 years.

The column labeled "Materials" is optional as a separate column. You can include this information in the activities column or separate it as you choose. If you do this separately, then you can include the names of the materials, the location, etc., here instead of on a back page. It is really up to you. One consideration is the page readability: The more columns you add, the less space to write in each column, and narrow columns are more difficult to read. I like to attach an original, very clean copy of any handout or game sheet to the back of the plan at this point. There is nothing more frustrating than going to produce handouts and finding out that your sheet is so old or perhaps a tenth-generation copy that it will not duplicate clearly.

Another consideration is the formatting needed when submitting your lesson plan to an accrediting body for continuing education credits. You will find that the format I use is also used by most agencies, and when you receive a form to complete to obtain continuing education units (CEUs), the format of the lesson plan may look exactly like, or close to, this lesson plan. It has become fairly standard over the years.

The last column requests that you identify the instructor. You may feel that it is unnecessary or redundant when you teach all the classes, but think about it. If you are team teaching the class, the plan will tell you who teaches each subject or objective. It is perfectly acceptable to identify the instructor by title or discipline rather than by name. If you are applying for CEUs, you must name and include the curriculum vitae (resume) for each instructor.

The lesson plan is now complete. Great job!

I suggest that, the first time you teach this class, you ask another instructor to sit in the class and check the lesson plan step-by-step as you go. Encourage the reviewer to write notes on the plan and fill in the content that you have missed. Actually, it is a lot more common that you are teaching additional content not listed on the lesson plan. It helps to know that, too, so you can thoroughly document your lessons. Your reviewer might want to make suggestions for things to include in the program and correct the time frame for the topics, as it never works out as planned the first time.

This means that your original lesson plan is always a draft. Of course. A class or a course is a living, breathing thing and grows and develops as you grow, develop, and mature. It is exciting and sometimes amusing to go back and look at the lesson plans from years back. Here is one of my old ones. I thought you might enjoy it. It was written in 1975, after I first learned to do this stuff. Bad, right? *See Lesson Plan A.*

Could you step in and teach this class for me? Probably not. Do you see how the content of three lines will be covered in 75 minutes?

Lesson Plan B is a sample of a wonderful lesson plan for a patient education class developed by Mary Lemesevski, ARNP, MSN, CDE, at Valley Hospital in Ridgewood, NJ, a former colleague. See how detailed and complete it is? Could you take this lesson plan and teach this class? Of course. Note that Mary's plan has no time frame so she can adjust the time spent in the course based on the assessed needs of the learners in that class, which she does at the beginning of the course.

Lesson Plan C is one of my lesson plans that has nothing to do with diabetes. It is a workshop on customer satisfaction. I conduct it for nursing homes and hospitals and have a great time. Think it might be fun to teach?

I had a family emergency once and had to miss a workshop that I was to conduct at Joslin Clinic in Boston. I was devastated but really had no choice. Fortunately, a wonderful colleague happened to be visiting Joslin that day and was asked to help out by conducting my course. This was a five-hour workshop. Imagine that: She had never seen the program but was an expert in the field. She was given my lesson plans and participant handouts and went on to do that program with great success. She met all the objectives, and the learners were able to get all of the information, skills, and knowledge that I had intended to give them if I taught the course myself. Did they get the stories and analogies that I use?

Lesson Plan A

Objectives	Content (Topics)	Time Frame	Faculty	Teaching Method
List objectives in operational/behavioral terms.	List each topic area to be covered and provide a description or outline of the content to be presented.	State the time frame for the topic area.	List the faculty person or presenter for each topic.	Describe the teaching method(s) used for each.
At the conclusion of this offering, participants will be able to	I. Patient education as a living, breathing thing a. definition of adult learning and patient education b. the Do-Know-Deficit	60 minutes	Ginger S. Kanzer, RN, EdM, CDE (resume attached)	Lecture/discussion, overhead/slides
1. define adult and patient education				
2. explain the Do-Know-Deficit	II. Why me? I have enough to do! a. the role of the staff nurse in patient education b. how to fit education in when you are working c. the staff nurses' role vs. the educator's role	30 minutes		
3. discuss the role of staff nurses in patient education and why they do not consider it a priority	III. OK! How do I do it? a. teaching learning techniques b. creating learning experiences on the units	75 minutes	Ginger S. Kanzer, RN, EdM, CDE	Lecture/discussion, overhead/slides
4. identify ways of dealing with teaching/learning problems	IV. How do I put it on paper? a. documentation skills b. forms and format c. legal ramifications of patient education	75 minutes		
5. discuss the documentation and accountability of patient education	V. Dealing with learning problems a. handling the family b. patients with special problems c. the non-compliant patient	45 minutes		
6. discuss effective and efficient ways to document	VI. Putting it all together a. summation b. questions and answers	35 minutes	Ginger S. Kanzer, RN, EdM, CDE	Lecture/discussion, overhead/slides
7. identify the legal ramifications involved with documentation of patient education				

Of course not, but they knew what I wanted them to know by the end of the session, and I wasn't even there. Thanks, Carelyn Fylling, MSN, RN, for saving the day!

Completing lesson plans for each of your classes will give you an extra marketing tool for the programs you conduct for colleagues and health care professionals. Once you're completely comfortable with the process and do it quickly and easily, you will find that you now have most of the application for CEUs. You are then able to give the staff in your own facility credits for attending your in-house programs. It is a great incentive to increase attendance and a wonderful motivating tool. It will also impress your boss and facility that you are capable of doing this—and that doesn't hurt.

Lesson Plan D is a blank curriculum form from the American Association of Diabetes Educators (AADE). This is the form you must complete if you submit an application for CEUs to AADE. The columns should look very familiar.

Lesson Plan B

Title of Offering: What Is Diabetes?   **Goal:** Recognition of Health Problem

Content	Objectives	Activities	Resources	Evaluation

1. Define diabetes
2. Normal metabolism
  a. glucose metabolism
  b. normal blood glucose
     levels
	All the completion of this session, the learning will be able to
	
	1. Define diabetes mellitus
	
	2. Describe normal physiology of food metabolism
		Discussion
		Transparencies
		Video
			"A CORE CURRICULUM FOR DIABETES EDUCATION" 2nd ed. American Assoc. of Diabetes Educators
			V. Peragallo-Dittko, RN, MA, CDE
			J. Godley, RN, MS, CDE
			J. Meyer, RN, MSN, FAAN, CDE
			
			Video: "Understanding your Diabetes"
			
			In Balance, In Control
			Boehringer Mannheim Corp.
				Discussion

3. Pathophysiology of diabetes
  a. food metabolism
  b. glucose metabolism
  c. types of diabetes mellitus
    (DM)
  d. causes of DM
  e. treatment of DM
	3. Describe the pathophysiology of diabetes	Discussion
		Transparencies
			RN
			Certified Diabetes Educator
				Discussion

4. Recognition of hypoglycemia and hyperglycemia a. cause	4. Define hypoglycemia and hyperglycemia	Discussion Transparencies	RN Certified Diabetes Educator	Discussion

5. Signs & Symptoms
  a. treatment
  b. record-keeping
	5. List the signs, symptoms, and treatment of hypoglycemia and hyperglycemia			

Lesson Plan C

Program Title: Customer Satisfaction   Speaker: Ginger Kanzer-Lewis, RNC, EdM, CDE

Program Learning Objectives	Program Topics	Program Content Outline	Time Frame	Teaching Method	Faculty
At the end of this presentation, the participant will be able to	Major content headings to accomplish objective	Subtopics or areas of detail and explanation of major content areas	Projected minutes per topic	Media, methods, materials used to present topic	
1. Discuss the purpose of the program, its focus, and scope	Purpose of program, focus, & scope	Why is a customer satisfaction necessary and important? Why is it necessary to change the culture of an organization in order to satisfy clients? Why are we starting this program with the nursing dept?	30 minutes	Lecture with PowerPoint; group discussion and brainstorming	Ginger Kanzer-Lewis, RNC, EdM, CDE
2. Identify who are the customers, internal and external	Identification of "customers"	Internal customers: patients, families, doctors, administrators, employees, volunteers & quality assurance/improvement committees External customers: 3rd-party reimbursement agencies, medicare, medicaid, accreditation agencies, vendors, health care agencies, home care agencies, etc.	30 minutes	Brain storming session	GKL

3. Identify what upsets patients and their families	What do your customers/clients want?	What do the internal customers want? Information, competency, knowledge, concern and caring What do external customers want? Quality care, low cost and satisfied customers Doing an assessment of your facility	90 minutes	Group discussion and brainstorming; presentation and film "It's a Dog's World"	GKL
4. Identify a plan of action to improve their scores	Developing a plan of action for their facility	What would you like to do in your facility? What exists now? Are you satisfied? What needs to be improved? How can it be improved? How far are you willing to go?	60 minutes	Small group work and reporting	GKL
5. Identify how to make customer satisfaction the culture of their facility	Changing the culture of their facility to be customer friendly	How to get the staff involved How to spread the news How to get all stakeholders involved How to conduct focus groups How to market the process	60 minutes	Group work and reporting; brainstorming; lecture with PowerPoint	GKL

Lesson Plan D

Program Title: _____ Speaker: _____

Program Learning Objectives	Program Topics	Program Content Outline	Time Frame	Teaching Method	Faculty
At the end of this presentation, the participant will be able to	Major content headings to accomplish objective	Subtopics or areas of detail and explanation of major content areas	Projected minutes per topic	Media, methods, materials used to present topic	
					Question and answer period
					Complete forms

10

Developing an Education Program

I would like to give you some cautions and suggestions that are not usually written in the how-to manuals.

So you want to develop an education program, perhaps a diabetes education program. Why?

That's the first question you need to answer. Doesn't one already exist in your area? Is the existing program overloaded or overwhelmed? Are you getting requests from endocrinologists or general practitioners in the area for help? Are patients contacting your facility and looking for a diabetes program? Are the patients in your area not being cared for or being taught well?

If you cannot answer these questions, why are you starting a program?

If the only reason for developing a program is that you are very interested in diabetes and want to teach it, consider your options. Can you join an existing program? Can you get involved with the local American Diabetes Association and volunteer your time to teach groups in the community? Can you teach patients in your own setting without setting up a formal cost center or a diabetes self-management education department?

If you are planning to do this because someone in your organization has discovered that diabetes education is now a reimbursable service under Medicare, Medicaid, and private insurance and thinks this is a new way to make money for the facility, you are in for a rude awakening. Over 1,000 diabetes programs have closed over the past two years because of reimbursement issues and the inability of the programs to produce the budgeted revenues or break even.

Does this mean that no new programs should be developed? Absolutely not, but they should be developed for the right reasons. I have had a sign in my office for many years. It says, "If you think education is expensive, try ignorance."

If you have investigated your area and identified that there is a need for a program that is not being met, go for it!

Now that you have done your "needs assessment," how do you start? Fortunately, you do not have to begin from scratch. If you decide to develop a diabetes education program, it would be foolish not to develop one that is "state-of-the-art," with the excellent resources available to you. There is a chapter in the *Core Curriculum for Diabetes Education* from the American Association of Diabetes Educators that takes you through the process and is great advice for the beginner. American Diabetes Association published the *National Standards for Diabetes Self-Management Education* (see References), which clearly list the components of a program and the expectations required if you plan to apply for Recognition. The American Diabetes Association publishes the *Diabetes Education & Recognition Resource*, which provides guidance on how to develop your program and achieve Recognition, step-by-step.

It is much easier to develop a program that meets the National Standards for Diabetes Self-Management Education right from the start than trying to adapt your program later when you decide it is time to apply for Recognition.

Investigate what resources already exist in your own organization, e.g., what is currently being done or is being planned by another department or group of people. Many years ago, I decided to develop a COPD education program and identified a grant that was available from the local office of the American Lung Association. I gathered all my information and was deep into the application process when I happened to mention to a colleague what I was doing. He asked whether my work was part of the program that the respiratory therapy department was developing. When I decided to talk to the head of respiratory therapy, I discovered that they had done a survey of the area, submitted a proposal to the hospital administration, and put many of the steps in place. They did not think it necessary to contact the education department, and I did not contact them. We both missed the boat. When we collaborated on the program, we developed a very successful, funded program that the patients, physicians, and administration loved and is still in place 20 years later.

Lest you think that I am the only naiive person in education, here is a fun story. I was invited to the Walter Reed Army Medical Center in Washington, DC, to conduct my "Patient Education: Just Do It!" workshop for the nursing administrative group—the directors, managers, head nurses, etc. There were to be about 200 people in this large medical center. I arrived the day before and decided to conduct an assessment with the colonel who had invited me, who was establishing a patient education department. He had told me that there was little, or no, patient education being done, and the staff at the center were committed to learning and moving forward. I requested a tour of the facility, and what a learning experience it was. On each unit, I asked the nurse manager what was being taught to patients about their specialty, and almost without fail, they explained their program and in many cases showed me the cardiac, orthopedic, or diabetes manual the staff had developed. The colonel was astounded. When I asked whether they were sharing the manuals throughout the organization or publishing their materials for the educators in other army hospitals (or even for civilians), they were surprised. Many of their materials were excellent for professionals or patients alike. I was very impressed and used their tools as illustrations during my program the next day. Interesting? **They had done all this wonderful work and never shared or published it.**

Find out who would be your best support and biggest antagonists in creating your education program. In the beginning, it was very difficult, because I had to justify my program to almost everyone. Because of what we have learned about the importance of education in health outcomes, this is not the issue it was years ago, but there are still people who will be concerned that you are interfering with their practice or "stealing their patients." These may be general practitioners who still hesitate to refer patients to specialists for the same concerns.

There are a few things I would suggest.

Create an advisory board. When you establish your Patient Education Advisory Board, a requirement of the National Standards for Diabetes Self-Management Education, think about who you ask to serve. You will, of course, want to include your greatest supporters, physicians who believe the program will improve the lives of people with diabetes and who will utilize and refer to your program. The other function of these wonderful doctors is to represent you and your program at medical board meetings, medical staff meetings, and continuing education programs. They will be your strongest advocates and give you guidance and assistance of great value.

On the other hand, I sometimes ask my most verbal antagonist to serve on the board. I had a physician early on who insisted that I would be going to jail for practicing medicine without a license. I had our medical director ask him to join the group, and he became a great supporter. (I think this move kept me out of jail.)

Your advisory board is made up of people with expertise in all of the disciplines that are involved in patient education and who are great resources for you and your department. Please do not forget to include a patient or patients on the board. It is a requirement, but more important, they are valuable advisors. With their guidance, you might avoid some of the mistakes health care professionals make when they are the only decision makers for patients.

I highly recommend that you have a Patient Education Advisory Board rather than a separate group for diabetes education, unless you know that you will only be teaching people with diabetes. Most of us start off with a limited scope and expand our horizons. People are not just parts and often have comorbidities. You will get into cardiac education, respiratory education, exercise, smoking cessation, weight control, etc. Why limit your education to one category of people? You will see it keeps growing and expanding. It's fascinating.

Identify your clients and territory. Who will you teach? When will you teach them? Where will you teach? Don't laugh. Classroom space is always at a premium and may be difficult to come by. Audiovisual equipment can be expensive, and you absolutely need it. I have had to teach a patient to inject insulin in the back of the chapel because someone was using my classroom for a meeting. Is there going to be a private area for you to talk to patients, with or without their families?

Do the math. Have you ever had to develop a budget for a department? What is this whole thing going to cost? Really. Talk to the chief financial officer and financial staff and ask them what kind of information they will need from you before they set up a cost center. What will be the expenses, and what revenue are you projecting? Talk to the education department if one exists in your facility. Talk to another department that provides comparable services for patients, e.g., physical therapy, and find out how they do their billing.

Develop an action plan. From the moment you get the idea for an education program, until the ribbon-cutting ceremony, there will a time frame. Think it out, and work it out. Don't make promises you cannot keep. There are so many things that need to be done getting started that you should not underestimate the work required.

Don't do work that has already been done. For diabetes, the Standards tell you the content areas that must be included. Programs have been developed and are available for purchase that will wind up being much cheaper, if purchased and adapted to your setting, than if you start from scratch. You can find wonderful curricula and guidelines.

Set up a documentation system. There are all kinds of options, and if you are fortunate enough to be able to set up a computer diabetes management system from the beginning, you will be way ahead of the game. I am biased, however, as I have been working on a software program for three years with a wonderful company and know the benefits.

Find a management sponsor. Find the person in your organization, large or small, who is very interested and willing to serve on your advisory board. That person will advocate for you with the most important people. They will speak for you in administrative meetings and find the funds to support the program. Bless these people.

Set up a marketing plan. Find the person in your organization who is most capable of marketing and can advise and assist you in this process. Every time you do something for the community, make sure you get publicity. Find every way you can to get your department or yourself in the local papers. Do health fairs and public relations events. Your boss will love opening the paper and seeing the program highlighted. Remember, it is harder to fire you or close your department if the Chamber of Commerce just gave you an award.

Do the research. For diabetes, I suggest the journal *The Diabetes Educator*, published by the American Association of Diabetes Educators, as a great resource on developing a program and avoiding the pitfalls.

I cannot address all the things you will need to do to establish an education department or program, but following my suggestions might make your life a little easier. Good luck and have fun!

11

Teaching Health Care Professionals to Teach

There is absolutely no point in asking health care providers to teach anything at all, unless you are prepared to teach them how to do it and motivate them to want to teach.

We tell people to teach and expect them to do it but are always surprised when it is not done, or not done well. Teaching is part of the scope and standards of practice of all health care providers, but it was not until the last decade that professional schools of health care began to include the teaching of patients in their curricula. The reality is that the nursing profession has a lot more middle-aged people in clinical practice than young staff, and some were not taught how to teach patients.

I addressed the other issue previously: adding more work to the workload of the overburdened staff. How can you expect them to add patient education to their list of daily activities?

First, teach them how to teach. All professional staff at my hospital, 1,300 RNs and 2,700 employees, were expected to attend the all-day session on which this book is based. Sometimes that meant I had to offer it once a month. Every other month, I ran an evening class or a weekend session to accommodate the diverse schedules.

The session was eight hours long and awarded CEUs, so the nursing and dietary staff were given an extra bonus for attending. The hospital made a commitment that it would be part of all staff responsibility and made the choice to pay the staff for attending. Fortunately, this was an affluent hospital whose decision makers felt the program was part of their commitment to quality.

To fund the program, we submitted an application for a grant to our own development department. This is the hospital's foundation, which raises money for worthwhile causes and seeks funding for specific projects that would be considered too expensive for the operating budget. We were fortunate to have such a funding resource, something not feasible for all facilities. This project was underwritten by a three-year grant. It was very exciting.

However, could you find some way to update your staff in educational methodology without breaking the bank? If you want people to teach, you need to give them the tools.

In the beginning, we kept all diabetes education materials in the nursing education department and brought them to class or to the units as necessary or when requested. We then found that there were patients admitted when we were off duty or on vacation. Calls at home from frustrated nurses forced us to identify a gap in our customer service.

Mary Lemesevski, ARNP, MSN, CDE, came up with a great idea. We bought fishing tackle boxes for each unit and equipped them with everything we wanted the nurses to use when teaching a patient. This included all the handouts and paperwork we would use, but we added more things to the box. There were now meters, strips, lancets, and logbooks. We added saline and syringes and all the teaching tools a staff nurse might need to teach a patient in our absence. We took the frustration and the time-consuming task of putting things together out of the equation. Just having teaching manuals and documentation forms all in one spot diminished the burden of teaching. No longer could people offer us the excuse that they could not teach a person self-monitoring of blood glucose because they did not have a meter for a demonstration.

Weekly, we checked the boxes and replaced any missing materials. The way we looked at it, the more we had to replace, the more that had been taught. It was very exciting.

We also developed the documentation tools to cut down on the charting. Assessment sheets and flow sheets contained the data we needed without requiring reams of narrative notes in the chart. It was easy to document with check-off forms.

We also offered them a support structure. We identified a group of nurses who would be part-time diabetes teaching nurses. These were people who would like to become certified diabetes educators (CDEs) but needed the skills, experience, and practice in order to meet the requirements. You must have 1,000 clinical hours of diabetes self-management education experience within the past five years to sit for the National Certification Board for Diabetes Educators examination.

These nurses were regular staff nurses who worked on the clinical units and devoted one day a week to the diabetes education department. We paid them on a per-diem basis, and they became wonderful educators. Because several of them worked the evening or night shift, they became available as a resource to the entire hospital while on duty. It worked out well for everyone and created a wonderful support structure.

I often met with them for short conference sessions and gave them teaching suggestions and adult education methodology. They attended Mary's or my classes, and we modeled adult education for them. They team-taught our evening group sessions with us, and I am pleased to say, several of them now work full-time as CDEs.

Teach people to teach, and they will reach a comfort zone that will take the fear out of teaching. Remember, surveys say that pubic speaking is more feared by people than dying.

Now that you taught them how to teach, teach them what to teach. When you read Chapter 12 on building the new team, you will understand the importance of educating the entire community. You need to be able to state what you have done for your own people.

When was the last time you conducted diabetes update classes for your own staff? Do you attend workshops and seminars and keep the information to yourself? Have you found a wonderful chart on the actions of insulins and not posted it in every medication room in the clinic or on the nursing stations of the local hospital? I know you bring all your friends toys from the conventions you attend, but do you bring back and hang up posters and signs that say, "Before you see the doctor, take off your shoes and socks!"?

Are you comfortable showing a medical colleague the latest article on pumps or the islet cell surgery being done in Canada? Are you the only one receiving continuous education on diabetes in your facility?

Sharing your knowledge will only add to our patients' knowledge and skills and might even lighted your burden. I know you want to be all things to all people, but do a reality check. Are you doing too much because there is no one to help you, or is there no one to help you because you have not shared your knowledge and skills? Think about it.

12

Building a Patient Education Environment and the New Team

I believe if the patient is to benefit, we need to develop health care without walls or barriers.

I have been developing diabetes education programs for many years and including educators from all disciplines. Early on, I discovered that people in other specialties could contribute expertise and experience to the courses and help improve the lifestyle of people with diabetes.

This became evident early on when the new species, diabetes educators, discovered that the learner often needed more materials and subject matter than we were comfortable delivering. Most of the early diabetes educators, or people who started teaching people with diabetes, were nurses. I like to call them "puffs," not to be confused with the brand name of tissues.

Someone in administration noticed that you were teaching patients, or were good at teaching staff, or worked in staff development or in nursing education, or were a dietitian who identified a patient with a health care learning need. The administrator turned to you and waved his magic wand. Puff! You were now in patient education. Wonderful. Many of you got to go into the new role and kept your other job in addition. Do you wear many hats?

I have never been a full-time diabetes or patient educator. For the last 30 years, I have been director of inservice, staff development, community education, patient education, etc., and have never held the title of diabetes educator. Interesting, huh?

Somewhere along the way, I found a colleague who was interested in what I was trying to do and asked her to join in. I was lucky enough to find Liz Kennett, BSN, RN (and now CDE), in New Hampshire, and she is still running the diabetes program at Catholic Medical Center 30 years later.

When nurses discovered how much diet meant to the new diabetics, as they were called in those days, and how complex the "diabetic diets" were, we needed to solicit the help and knowledge of the dietitians. Here was a bright, caring group of people who were not called upon often by nurses in nonteaching facilities. Community hospitals had administrative dietitians to help food service departments plan the "special diets" for patients. When I consulted my friend Mary Austin, MA, RD, CDE, for her memory of the early days, she said that the majority of diabetes nutrition education was done while the patient was hospitalized or, more likely, just before the patient was being discharged. She recalls teaching many "ADA diet" instructions as the patient was fully dressed, packed, and ready to go out the door. Nurses faced the same challenge when teaching insulin injection and other self-care skills. Sending patients to regularly scheduled inpatient or outpatient diabetes classes was a solution to a frustrating situation for dietitians, nurses, and patients alike. Teaming up with a nurse only made sense.

In 1993, the Diabetes Complications and Control Trial[18] clearly identified that the most effective approach to improving

[18] DCCT study. See References.

the quality of care of people with diabetes was a multidisciplinary approach.

Mulcahy[19] identified the components of the diabetes team. To meet American Diabetes Association standards, you must include an RN and an RD on your diabetes team. The coordinator of the program should be a CDE, and the RN has three years from this point to become a CDE in order to be coordinator of the program. We have identified that although these people are certainly competent to teach a diabetes education program, there are more great resources who should be included.

The Old Health Care Team

- Made up of people
- People represented the health care disciplines
- Sometimes people had vested interests or personal agendas
- They worked for a specific organization or company
- They did "snap shot" teaching

Who better than a pharmacist is qualified to teach about medications? Which social worker would not be an asset when talking about family issues or lifestyle changes? Perhaps a psychologist could become involved to discuss the depression and support circles involved in living a life with diabetes? You may not be able to get Terry Saunders, PhD, or Richard Rubin, PhD, for your team, but there have got to be wonderful people in your area.

What exercise program could not benefit from the contributions of a physical therapist or an exercise physiologist? Please don't forget that the physician is always part of the team, and find the best support you can for your program. You are required to have a medical director for the program, and he or she becomes such an asset when it comes to advocating for your program with

---

[19] Mulcahy K: Architects of the diabetes team. See References.

the medical staff. The list can go on, and if anyone is feeling left out, I invite them to join my team.

There is another issue about team building that is very urgent to me. I call it the "new team" concept.

The "old team" is and was wonderful, but there were some issues at times. The old team was made up of people who represented their disciplines and sometimes were territorial or had their own agendas. They worked for a specific organization or company and had goals that were sometimes set by the organization. Materials and programs were developed for that organization and became the property of the organization. Competition was sometimes mandated, and although many of us had no difficulty sharing ideas or materials, it was sometimes politically incorrect. I remember sharing materials with the educator across town, but my administrator would not have been happy if he had known about it.

We don't need to put up roadblocks to education; it only hurts our patients. Patients are more demanding, and the health care system is changing. Reimbursement is changing and is not the universal panacea we expected it to be when we helped pass the legislation. Patients are more curious. They are information sponges, and if they cannot get the information they want from you, they will use all their resources to search for the answer they want. I have seen patients come to class with computer printouts of my resume and even a picture from my web site.

The New Health Care Team

- Made up of people, facilities, and groups
- Creates heath care without walls:
  - All health care disciplines included
  - All types of agencies included
- Creates consistency for patients:
  - Everyone talks the same language
  - Centers on common concerns
  - Forms a solid circle of support

The new team is broader. It includes multiple facilities and groups. Instead of a multidisciplinary group of people, it is a community-wide group of facilities that are grouped together to meet the needs of people with diabetes. Each group needs a hub; I see that being the acute care setting, hospital, clinic, or medical group that has the original multidisciplinary group of primary care providers. Often this is the entry site for the patient and where the initial diagnosis occurs.

The new team creates health care without walls. All disciplines are included, and all types of agencies are involved. It creates consistency for patients, with everyone talking the same language. Everyone has common concerns, and it eliminates confusion while creating a solid circle of support.

How is this done? Can the primary diabetes program take on the responsibility of training the staff of all facilities in the community? Think about these and the following questions. I don't always have the answers, but I ask great questions.

When you send a child home from your program, have you educated the school nurses and the teachers in his school? Are they prepared to accept and assist this child in his environment? Last year, a school principal pulled an insulin pump off a child because he thought it was a pager. This is an example of a horrible outcome that's due to not educating everyone about the child and his pump.

Do you hold classes for grandparents, even babysitters, for the family of children? Who helps those people become support for those overwhelmed parents?

What about the nursing home staff who care for the elderly patient whom you transferred back after a hospital stay? Have you held diabetes update classes for their staff before there is a problem with your patient? I have been consulting for a group of nursing homes. I did an audit in one facility; 40 of their 60 patients who are insulin treated are still getting one dose of NPH per day. I had a long discussion with their medical director and did a short inservice (education class) for their nursing staff.

What about the visiting nurses, public health staff, and home nurses in your area? Have you given a diabetes therapy update recently for their people? What is the sense of teaching patients in a hospital and/or clinic and sending the patient home with a referral for follow-up care when the provider uses different languages or even contradicts your advice or information? Remember that "little bit of sugar" stuff? There are lots of new medications that may be news to this group, which has to know so much about all kinds of patients.

Have you brought the pharmacists in your area together for a short meeting to discuss the current trends in diabetes care? Do they know what meters you recommend so they keep them in stock? Do they know the current reimbursement issues for strips and meters? Many patients are spending or losing money because heath care providers do not know the steps they must take to help their patients get reimbursed. So, the patients have to pay out of pocket.

How about presenting a CEU program for general practioners in your area? Would your endocrinologist join you in conducting a program for the medical staff in a local community hospital? It could net him more referrals as well as build a collegial relationship between you and the local physicians.

Have you worked with your county public health department? They have resources for you and have established channels for getting the message out to the community about this important health care resource. I worked on several task forces with the New Jersey Public Health Department and had input when they set their goals and priorities for the year. I worked with wonderful people from many diverse agencies and learned a great deal about planning for a community.

This seems like a lot of work? What are the benefits?

Everyone talks the same language and stops confusing the patients. They become the center of the team and feel a part of the decision-making group.

We can establish goals and measure outcomes. When we all know the plan of action and the intention of the plan, you have a stronger commitment to assist the patient in keeping to the plan. This will help eliminate the covert saboteurs, the well-meaning people who want to help but haven't a clue that they are obstructionist when they tell the patient to just avoid concentrated sweets.

We update and educate professionals. We have documentation that less than 10% of people with diabetes see diabetes educators or endocrinologists. It then makes it essential that we contribute to the knowledge of the people who are actually seeing these people.

We satisfy patients and families. They are more confident when they believe their health care providers are competent in the field and that a communication network exists between their health care specialists.

We satisfy accrediting agencies. When they survey your program and see the commitment to patient care and the support you are providing your clients, they are very pleased. These relationships meet the patient education requirements from the Joint Commission on Accreditation of Healthcare Organizations.

We satisfy managed care agencies. Their goal is quality care at low costs, and when their beneficiaries are given good care at good prices, they are much more apt to negotiate better contracts with your facility.

We satisfy professional concerns. Meeting the requirements of professional associations for continuing education to earn CEUs gives all of us an opportunity for growth and development.

The present is driving the future of health care and patient education. The advent of new technologies is driving the system. New medications, meters, pumps, and surgical techniques require more sophisticated education and the expansion of team relationships.

> ## Choose to Keep Up!
>
> - New medications
> - New technologies: meters, pumps, tests
> - New surgical techniques
> - New research
> - New teamwork
>
> - New systems:
>   - Outcomes studies
>   - Managing patient with data, not guessing
>   - Disease management
>   - Research-driven practice
>   - Translation of research

In all health care fields, there is new research that opens opportunities for new teamwork.

There are new systems that require the expansion of the team. Outcomes studies have proven that the team is more effective than any one discipline. We are into disease management and evidence-based practice. We are translating the research into clinical practice, and it takes all kinds of people in all kinds of settings to do the work that used to be much more limited.

And, finally, will you fit into the new team? Have you acquired the skills and knowledge to meet with these people as a patient advocate? Can you convince your administration that expanding your team to the community is within your scope of practice and the right thing to do? Have you the political savvy to find the funding for this expansion in this constrained funding environment? Have you the marketing skills to sell this idea to the people who need to be sold on it? How are you going to convince the school system to let you in?

It's a big job, and whether it's diabetes, HIV/AIDS, or multiple sclerosis, we can no longer limit our roles to the four walls of our offices and classrooms. Good luck!

13

Marketing Your Program and Finding Funding

Because many health care organizations are still nonprofit, intentional or not, let's discuss finding funds for them.

Whether you have just developed a program or work in an established department of long-standing, someone is going to sit you down to discuss paying for it. No matter how much value you bring to the community and how committed your organization is to maintaining the program, funding is always an issue and needs to be a planned component of your proposal and annual plan.

Can you exist on your operating budget, or do you need to seek funding from different sources? When budget time comes in organizations, they ask for input from department heads; then they have to make difficult decisions, because resources only go so far and the organization has diverse goals.

Ask yourself the following questions. Should you seek funding? Does your facility consider this part of your job, or does it have a person responsible for this? Is there a development department or a foundation attached to the organization? Are you a nonprofit or profit-making organization? It is almost impossible to get grants and donations if yours is a for-profit facility, but there are some things you can do.

Should you seek internal or external funding? Some hospitals and outpatient clinics belong to a large hospital conglomerate. There are major medical centers formed by the affiliation of five or six hospitals, often connected to a major university. Universities often have large endowments, yet it is rare that individual departments of the affiliated hospitals apply for a grant from their own foundation. Are you allowed to write an internal proposal to the university development office to fund a new project?

What if you have developed a patient education manual for cardiac care and need to print 10,000 copies for the next two years? You get estimates on printing and all the other work involved and predict that it will cost $25,000 to have these books printed. You discuss it with your department head, and they say the funds are just not there for next year. What do you do? The first question should be, if I can find the money, can we do it? If the answer is "yes," and it will be, here are some suggestions.

First, make sure you have accurately predicted the costs. Never mind what it cost last year; costs go up constantly. The worst thing that can happen is that you get the $25,000 and find out the final costs are $26,000, and you are short. Are you going to put the rest of the money up yourself?

Develop a cost estimate and list all the direct and indirect costs. Some budget managers insist that you add in employees' time, electricity, copy machine costs, and mailing as well as the direct cost of printing the manual.

Then you need to write a proposal. Be clear. What do you want to do? Why do you want to do it? Is this new material, or does it replace something else? How many will you print, and how long do you expect that supply to last? If you get funding and print a two-year supply of books, what are you going to do after that, when the money is gone and you have no books left? Finally, why should any organization give you money? How will it benefit

Where to Find the Funds

- Your organization:
  - Grants
  - Restricted funds
  - Patient gifts
- Health care organizations
- Foundations and philanthropic agencies
- Industry
- Federal government
- State government
- County or local government

them? Will they receive publicity, a plaque, or a sign on the door of the classroom?

We are all altruistic at times and do things because they are right and good and make sense. Then there is the real world. I work with many of the large pharmaceutical companies, and they are wonderful and very generous with their time and money. When I was president of the American Association of Diabetes Educators, these companies made my projects happen—they could not have been done without the generous support of these companies. The question they always ask, however, is, "Why should we support this project and not another?" They were and are entitled to the answer. So are the people you contact for funding.

Who can you ask for money? Internally, look for grants, restricted funds, patient gifts, state health department funding, and county funds. Often, patients or relatives of deceased patients will donate money to the hospital. We are not allowed to accept tips, but this is always a nice bonus when it happens. Can these gifts or restricted funds be used for your project?

Externally, federal, state, and local governments sometimes have funds for certain types of investigations or projects. Make it your business to discover what is available or what kinds of proposals seek funding each year. Have you ever spoken to local groups such as the United Way or the Rotary Club? In the early 1980s, I received a $15,000 grant from the United Way to attempt to computerize our diabetes programs records. It paid for our computer and a person to put in the data. Money isn't the only resource: Many large corporations have a "loan an executive program." Once you have identified that you need a person with a certain expertise to help you with a project, they will find the right person for you within their organization and pay his or her salary for several months while that person works for you. IBM did exactly that for one year to help us develop a marketing program for our patient education department.

Can you find philanthropic agencies or local or national pharmaceutical companies that might be interested in helping to print your book? Maybe they will let their publishing department edit the book or create the graphics free of charge.

A word of caution: Do not compete with other departments for the same grant or funding source. Before you submit anything to anybody, find out whether someone else in the organization is doing the same thing and make some decisions. Can you partner or piggyback onto their application? If they are asking for $400,000, and you add $25,000 to it, it will not seem as big a deal as a separate $25,000 application. The government does it all the time.

To find out what foundations exist and what money is available that year, visit the local library. There you will find a foundation directory, foundation grant index, and a book of foundation grants to individuals. The library will also have listings of local or regional grant sources. Most of this information can now be found online. In New York, we have the Foundation Center on 5th Avenue that is more than willing to help you.

The Federal Government has several directories:

- The *Catalog of Federal Domestic Assistance* (www.cfda.gov)
- The *Federal Register*
- *Federal Grants and Contracts Weekly*
- The *Resource Guide to Federal Funding*
- *U.S. Government Manual*

State sources include:

- Directory of State Grant Agencies
- State legislative newsletter

When you seek help from corporations, take care to identify the correct department. Believe me, they are not thrilled when they find out that you are talking to the wrong people in the wrong department and getting money from the wrong budget.

A successful grant proposal will contain the following information:

- **Summary:** Provide an overview of the project. What are you going to wind up with?
- **Introduction:** Who are you? Establish credibility. Point out what is in it for them. Are you asking for the whole amount, or are you looking for funds that your organization will match? This is very helpful—people are more apt to give you money if you are paying part yourselves and just need assistance.
- **Justification:** Establish why you need to do this project and/or why your clients need you to do this project. Document with facts, not guesses. People love numbers, and some want every little detail. (This is difficult for people like me who are not detail oriented and had to learn to satisfy the obsessive-compulsive people.) Did you do your needs assessment? What data do you have to present?
- **Objectives:** You need to be able to measure the outcomes of your project.
- **Methods:** What activities will you do to fulfill this project? What procedures must be taken?
- **Assessment:** How will you evaluate the project? Is it as simple as printing books and giving them to patients over the next two years?
- **The future:** What will happen to your project after funding ends?

- **Budget:** List your personnel, materials, and direct and indirect expenses.
- **Appendix:** Place letters of support from interested parties here. Can you get patients to write a letter about how the information in the handmade manual helped them, how much more accessible the information would be as a bound booklet, and how every patient needs one?
- **Title page:** Make it attractive and complete. They cannot give you money if they cannot locate you. Spelling does count! I once wrote a $6 million dollar proposal to a state that was funded, but they requested in the notification letter a copy without typos. I was so embarrassed!

There are ways to find the funds for things you want to do. It takes time, but you can get help. How about asking a large corporation to lend you their proposal writer to help you write some grants. Why not?

14

A Patient's Perspective

Here is an opportunity to look at the joy and frustrations of teaching patients.

This chapter is about the people we care for, in my case people with diabetes. It is stories about incidents that have occurred over the years. Several of the stories have been previously published on the web site www. DiabetesinControl.com., which is aware that they would be included in this book. In several cases, I will update you on the patient's condition and his or her life status. I have also asked a few of my patients and friends to comment on their experiences. Enjoy!

A Tale of Two Women

I would like to tell you a story about two women whom I shall call Tara and Sara. I met them recently in Florida, and they are originally from New York, just as I am. They are very interesting, bright, articulate women and represent two of the types of people with diabetes that I have taught most of my career.

Both are retired, professional women in their late 60s who were college educated. Both are still married to very pleasant, caring men and have children and grandchildren. They happen to be sisters-in-law. Both have a comfortable life that they have earned and deserve. Both are charming and lots of fun. Both have type 2 diabetes.

Tara is very concerned with her diabetes and is determined to be in the best condition and heath status for the rest of her life. I met her at the swimming pool exercising. She walks two to five miles every day, takes her insulin faithfully, and checks her blood glucose four times a day. She gets upset with peaks and valleys and tries to keep her glucose levels as close to normal as possible. She is a partner with her endocrinologist, whom she travels two and a half hours to see, and asks and reads about everything. She will attend any class or support group available. Lest you think that she is a "professional diabetic," know that she has a very rich, full life. She and her husband are wonderful dancers. Lest you think her a saint, know that she likes to eat rich desserts at dances. She thinks I don't notice. Now that we are friends, she has included me in her team. It is my pleasure.

Sara introduced herself to me as the "other type of diabetic." She is rather overweight and does not exercise at all. She tests her blood "sometimes, when I remember" and is somewhat embarrassed to say that to me. I never asked her. She told me that she is not a "real diabetic" because she does not take insulin. She said that she is not prepared to be a diabetic and has no real problems or complications with it—yet. At this point, she had gotten to me. I asked whether she had ever been to a class or taken a course on diabetes or been under the care of a diabetes educator? She took a class once a long time ago. It was not very interesting, she really couldn't get into it, and she couldn't remember the name of the educator. Her doctor made her go, and it really did not matter to her; after all, she is the other kind of diabetic.

Sound familiar? It made me sad to think of this really nice woman walking around in "diabetes limbo." I am concerned that we, diabetes educators and health care providers, somehow missed the boat with this lady. Somehow, we never found, or created, a teachable moment where we "gotchya." We did not turn her on to her own responsibilities and abilities or motivate her to want to care for herself. It is going to be much harder now.

Before we beat ourselves up completely, there is the other side of the coin. For many years, I believed that if a patient did not learn, then I had not taught correctly. I had failed and was a poor excuse for an educator. It took a long time for me to understand that education is a partnership and not just my job.

Sara is in denial. She does not want to be a "diabetic" or have to deal with it. She is a grown woman and has to make her own decisions and perhaps live with the ramifications. She is not ready to learn, and it may take a very long time for her to reach the stage where she needs to learn and wants some help. I may not see her again, and she was not at all interested in seeing the educator that I mentioned. When Bob Anderson and Marti Funnel talk about empowerment, they don't suggest you do it with a club or hold hostages. People need to control their own lives and destinies.

I assigned Tara and her husband to the case and hope they will wear Sara down or finally get to her. It was the best that I could do.

Recently, I saw Tara, and she is doing very well. She is on a new insulin regimen and doing much better with her lows. She has lost 30 pounds due to a major home move and some family stress and has no intention to lose more. She says it is fun to have a few pounds to gain. She looks wonderful and feels good. What about Sara? She is interested that Tara looks so good and may consider talking to her doctor about changing her medications. Small steps.

Patient Rights and Wrongs

I met a man in a nursing home in New York. He is a department head in the facility, where I was to teach a class that has nothing to do with diabetes. We were chatting about the course I would be teaching, and he asked me about my background. Naturally, the American Association of Diabetes Educators came into the conversation. That's when the whole discussion changed, a simple reminder that wherever we diabetes educators go, or whatever we do, diabetes cannot be left behind.

He told me about his beautiful two-year-old niece who had just been diagnosed with type 1 diabetes after an emergency experience in the hospital and how overwhelmed his brother and sister-in-law are. He spoke of the horror of the experience and said that although everyone was caring and kind, they really did not seem to know what to do to help this child and her family cope with the diagnosis and the life changes it would bring to this young family.

When I asked whether the family had been connected to a diabetes educator, he said "no." They had not been informed that such people exist. I asked whether the physician had referred them to a pediatric diabetes center, and the answer was again "no." At this point, I had to control my own anger and frustration that some health care providers had let this terrified family leave the hospital without a plan of action and the beginnings of a support system. How unfair that is, and indeed dangerous.

Although the parents had been taught by someone to test the toddler's blood and how to inject insulin, that was the limit of their education. No dietitian had seen them nor had they talked to a pediatric specialist or advanced nurse practitioner. No one had agreed to speak to other members of the family, including grandparents in acute distress and anguish. The parents were taking turns sitting at the child's bedside each night, afraid to leave her alone for fear that she would develop ketoacidosis or hypoglycemia.

Now, before you panic, please know that I connected them to a pediatric diabetes educator at a medical center near their home. They have made appointments to see all the people they need to receive help. I could not return home without finding resources for them that would enable them to sleep nights, but I am still angry.

We need to keep ringing the bell and pushing the concept of the patient's right to education. We need to believe that we can make a difference.

A pair of great educators, Betty Brackenridge, MS, RD, CDE, and Kris Swenson, RN, CDE, teach their patients about the little girl who is standing on the beach surrounded by starfish. She is throwing them back into the water one by one, when an adult asks her what she is doing. She says the starfish have been washed onto the shore and will die if they are not put back in the water. The adult laughs and says there are so many, how will you save them all? The little girl picks up a starfish and tosses it into the sea and looks at the grown person and says, "At least I saved that one." Thank you, Betty and Kris. You are both inspirations.

As I sit here looking at the sea full of starfish, I have to remember . . . one patient at a time.

I spoke to the nursing home department head a few months later. The family was involved with a pediatric endocrinologist and a team of diabetes educators. The family, including grandparents, aunts, uncles, and babysitters, have all been to education programs, and the family is doing well. They still have difficult times occasionally, but they are managing much better. Now that makes me smile.

Close to Home

A friend of mine, Bob, called and asked if he could come to my house to talk to me immediately. Of course, I said, come over now. He arrived in a panic. He had not been feeling well, and a friend of his, a person with diabetes for about a year, insisted on checking his blood sugar. It was 378 mg/dl before lunch. He was somewhat concerned, and I checked his blood sugar and found it was 525 mg/dl. Bob is an interesting man, very bright but somewhat unusual. He lives on a boat and works constantly as a private computer consultant. He does not have health insurance and has not been to a doctor for 10 years. He says he's healthy and had no need.

Bob had a terrible headache, looked pale, and did not have a doctor. I suggested that I take him to the emergency room. He refused, and I was in quite a quandary. He is an adult and in control but in an unsafe state in my house. We agreed that he would stay in my house that night and that I would check his fasting blood sugar in the morning. Then, we would decide what to do. One of us did not get much sleep that night, and it was not Bob. In the morning, his blood sugar was 350 mg/dl, and I convinced him to let me contact an endocrinologist friend of mine. He believed at this point that I was overreacting and that "it would go away" the next day. My colleague agreed to see him the next morning, and we agreed that I would do frequent blood testing that day and go to the ER if his blood sugar went above 500 mg/dl before the appointment. His urine tested small for ketones. That did not cheer me up much.

The next morning, he went to see my friend and was put on medication, etc. I took over the teaching and gave him a meter.

A month later, Bob was doing well. His fasting blood sugar was about 150 mg/dl, and he never went over 200 mg/dl. He lost five pounds and tests more than necessary. He exercises and watches everything he eats. I am somewhat encouraged, but he somehow believes that if he loses weight and gets his blood glucose down to normal, he won't have to take medication at all for the rest of his life. He certainly did not learn that from me. He's had small successes, but why is he so adamant about not being a diabetic?

Each person responds differently when given the news that he or she has diabetes. You now have a person who has been told she has a chronic disease that she will have to manage and live with for the rest of her life. She may have had a family member who had diabetes and developed complications. That person may have lost a leg or gone blind or wound up on dialysis from kidney failure.

People may not understand the word *diabetes* or the true implications and may have little or no knowledge of the condition at all. Sometimes, the situation is made worse if they have misinformation and/or believe the myths surrounding diabetes. They may not be willing or able to deal with the situation at all.

Where does that leave the concerned health care provider? Where can you start? What should you teach and when?

It has been my experience that patients go through the same five stages when told they have a chronic disease that Kubler-Ross identified in 1969 in her book *On Death and Dying* for people given a fatal diagnosis.

First, there is denial. They think, not me, it couldn't be me, I just have the flu or something. The lab work must be wrong, and you mixed me up with someone else. Mistakes happen all the time, and this is a mistake.

Second, they get angry. Why me? I am a good person. How about those drug dealers or criminals? It's not fair. I won't talk to you, Ginger. You don't know what you're doing.

Then they bargain, either with themselves, you, or perhaps God. I know what: I will lose the weight you told me to and get some exercise. I will even stop smoking, and then it will go away. You'll see.

Next, the depression comes, and they won't talk about it at all.

Finally, they reach the stage of acceptance and agree to deal with it. Then they are ready to learn. They may not accept it all or agree to everything, but until we can get them to this stage, it is very hard to motivate, educate, or help them.

They will go back and forth through these stages, and if they are fortunate, you as a health care provider will be willing to go through it with them.

Sometimes it will take months or even years for a patient to reach acceptance. During the course of their diabetes, they will respond to changes in their condition by reverting to an earlier stage or by asking for help from the support system they have built to help them manage their diabetes.

I have often found that a patient's response and progression through the above stages is directly tied to the manner in which the diagnosis was given. If the health care provider is clear, concise, and factual and gives the patient information and choices for success, he or she will respond differently than to the provider who is vague or makes the issue seem as if it's "no big deal." If the physician helps the patient make the decision to work with the entire health care team, the stages are not as long or difficult as when he or she has to go through them alone.

We need to become adept at identifying which stage the patient is presenting at each visit or at changes in his or her diabetic status. Too many of these patients get stuck in the depression phase, and this quite often goes undiagnosed. Working with your patients to identify the depression phase and knowing how to get them help will certainly improve their care. I suggest you read Richard Rubin, PhD, CDE, and colleagues' articles on depression and diabetes (see References).

I received the following letter and would like to share it with you. The "best friend" the writer is referring to is Bob in the story above. When I asked his permission to include it in the book, Courtland gave me permission to edit it. I would not change a word.

Dear Ginger,

As I look back on my own life, it is obvious that education has not influenced my understanding of how the body functions or my management of health. We are all told that we have to eat a balanced diet and get exercise, but so what? As my lifestyle changed from participation in sports and working in construction to business management, surprise has accompanied the health consequences.

As health problems have become too annoying to ignore, I have gone to the doctor. Without exception, the information received from the doctor was inadequate. It seems he can't be an educator because of time constraints. So, I have had to do research, ask questions, and try to ferret out what to do. When my blood pressure was measured at 160 over 95 and exercise was prescribed, it was a surprise and revelation to see it drop to a consistent 116 over 68. When it became unacceptable to feel mean and angry starting two hours after a meal, a change to a low-carbohydrate, high-protein diet with fruits and vegetables changed everything, so that I now enjoy a peaceful feeling all day with rare exception.

When my best friend became pale and almost passed out, and it hit me that he was drinking water continuously all day long, we measured his blood sugar level on a diabetic friend's machine; I saw numbers in the high 300s and called you. The management of his blood sugar level is based on a new education on how the body functions, and without your help and input this management would be woefully inadequate.

We go to the doctor for a checkup because we should or because of crisis. We leave okay or with a prescription. We certainly can't leave the office well educated as to *how our lifestyle affects our health*. It is very difficult to find information on what to do next. There should be a prescription for meaningful education and a follow-up.

The management of one's health should not begin in a crisis when damage is already done. Health education should be designed and made available so that more people are reached and then actually change their lifestyle to a healthy one. We should all be educated to react to changes in lifestyle that will damage our health, and we should be able to understand symptoms of problems that require a visit to the doctor.

Sincerely,
Courtland

Each patient's story is an education for the health care provider. We think we know what is best for patients and try to do all we can for all of them without considering their previous experiences with health care people. People with all kinds of diagnoses are treated well or treated badly because they come into contact with us, the professionals. I often ask nurses the following question: Are your patients better off because they met you today, or would they have been better off if you had called in sick and someone else had cared for them? That's a scary question. Think about it.

15

A Final Word—or Two

I developed a program called the "Diabetes World According to Me." It is a look at the future, and I would like to share it with you here.

Where do we go from here? We have looked at what patient education is and why we do it. We have gone through the components and how to do it step-by-step. We have talked about the patients, their successes, and our failures, but what is in the future?

The world has finally recognized that diabetes is an epidemic. The pulp magazines and respected new media are covering it weekly, and the government is making a commitment to deal with the concept of preventing diabetes with physical activity and weight control. The time for diabetes management may have arrived.

The health care world has discovered that diabetes educators make a difference. Christopher Saudek, MD, a past president of the American Diabetes Association, in his president's address stated that, "No diabetes management tool, no new oral agent, insulin, or medical device is as important as the services of a diabetes educator

(CDE). This relatively new health care professional has added immeasurably to the provision of good diabetes care . . ."

There has never been a better time to have diabetes and live well. There are new medications, new technology, new reimbursements, and a possible cure for diabetes hovering across the border in Edmonton, Canada. The future looks good. There are still more medications, including inhaled insulin, in the pipeline; new diagnostic tools; and new plans on the drawing boards.

More important, there are new attitudes toward diabetes. There may be more money, time, and energy directed toward something that affects so many people in the world that governments are setting up major incentives to deal with it. I am working on a major project with the government of Egypt for a 2003 presentation.

Unfortunately, some things remain the same. People all over the world are still dying. People are still not being treated correctly. People are still not being reimbursed properly and are having trouble paying for their care and supplies. People are still not being educated.

We have not convinced the public that this is a really serious disease. A wonderful colleague of mine, Richard Guthrie, MD, suggested years ago that we should put the shoes of all those who have lost their legs on the steps of the capitol in Washington, DC. Another colleague from Austria asked me why we still had so many diabetes-related cases of blindness in the United States when their numbers had been going down steadily for the past five years.

I frequently sit in meetings where we try over and over again to answer the question: How do we get the message out? For over 20 years, I have heard wonderful speakers at diabetes conventions all over the world, and still we preach to the choir.

How do we reach the primary care providers who are so very busy caring for patients that they cannot get to meetings? How do we reach the people who will not accept their diabetes and connect them with the people who can help them? How do we help the people we cannot reach?

Educators: Where to Go from Here

- The world has discovered that they need us.
- The opportunities are there for us to grow and change.
- We are the captains of our ships and the leaders of our futures.

Sounds like the never-ending story. I know how well people can do when they are connected to the right providers and educators. I have seen wonderful results, and the outcomes data have been coming in since the Diabetes Control and Complications Trial proved that patients do better with a team approach to diabetes care.

If the message sounds pessimistic, it is not. It is a call for awareness and a change to the thought process that believes that we have solved all the problems about diabetes care and education. As long as I cannot answer the why questions, we will be searching and looking and listening. So, I have some suggestions.

Let's start teaching everyone about diabetes, the entire public. Let's teach it in health classes in schools and to everyone who will listen. How about an information campaign about diabetes to people without diabetes? Maybe we will find those missing millions and get to the people who know the people with diabetes. The idea is to reach those people I meet on planes who tell me about friends and families. How about major radio and TV ads that do not target "diabetics" but ask whether the listener knows someone who has or may have diabetes? Perhaps we have been looking in all the wrong places?

Before you start throwing costs at me, I would like to remind you that the United States spent nearly $100 billion last year caring for people with diabetes. One in ten health care dollars is now spent on diabetes.

We can go forward. Our patients need us to push forward, and we can do it! I know we can. That's why I titled this book *Patient Education: You Can Do It!*

References and Suggested Reading

Ad Hoc Committee on Health Literacy for the Council on Scientific Affairs, American Medical Association: Health Literacy: Report of the Council on Scientific Affairs. *JAMA* 281: 552–557, 1999

American Association of Diabetes Educators: *AADE 2003 Member Resource Guide*. Chicago, American Association of Diabetes Educators, 2003

American Association of Diabetes Educators: *A Core Curriculum for Diabetes Education*. 4th ed. Chicago, American Association of Diabetes Educators, 2001

American Association of Diabetes Educators: Diabetes educational and behavioral research summit. *Diabetes Educ* 25 (Suppl.):2–88, 1999

American Diabetes Association: ADA Education Recognition Program. Available from *www.diabetes.org*. Accessed June 2000

American Diabetes Association: *Complete Guide to Diabetes*. 3rd ed. Alexandria, VA, American Diabetes Association, 2002

American Diabetes Association: *Diabetes Education Goals*. 3rd ed. Alexandria, VA, American Diabetes Association, 2002

American Diabetes Association: *Life with Diabetes: A Series of Teaching Outlines.* 2nd ed. Funnell MM, Arnold MS, Barr PA, Lasichak AJ, Eds. Alexandria, VA, American Diabetes Association, 2000

American Diabetes Association: National standards for diabetes self-management education (Standards and Review Criteria). *Diabetes Care* 26 (Suppl. 1): S149–S156, 2003

American Diabetes Association: Report of the Task Force on the Delivery of Diabetes Self-Management Education and Medical Nutrition Therapy. *Diabetes Spectrum* 12:44–47, 1999

Anderson B, Funnell M: *The Art of Empowerment: Stories and Strategies for Diabetes Educators.* Alexandria, VA, American Diabetes Association, 2000

Anderson B, Rubin RR (Eds.): *Practical Psychology for Diabetes Clinicians.* Alexandria, VA, American Diabetes Association, 2002

Anderson LA, Janes GR, Ziemer DC, Phillips LS: Diabetes in urban African Americans: body image, satisfaction with size, and weight change attempts. *Diabetes Educ* 23:301–308, 1997

Anderson RM: Patient empowerment and the traditional medical model: a case of irreconcilable differences? *Diabetes Care* 18:412–415, 1995

Anderson RM: The team approach to diabetes: an idea whose time has come. *Occup Health Nurs* 30:13–14, 1982

Anderson RM, Fitzgerald JT, Funnell MM: The diabetes empowerment scale (DES): a measure of psychosocial self-efficacy. *Diabetes Care* 23:739–743, 2000

Anderson RM, Funnell MM: Compliance and adherence are dysfunctional concepts in diabetes care. *Diabetes Educ* 2:597–604, 2000

Anderson RM, Funnell MM: The role of the physician in patient education. *Pract Diabetol* 9:10–12, 1990

Anderson RM, Funnell MM: Theory is the cart, vision is the horse: reflections on research in diabetes patient education. *Diabetes Educ* 25 (Suppl. 6):43–51, 1999

Anderson RM, Funnell MM: Using the empowerment approach to help patients change behavior. In *Practical Psychology for Diabetes Clinicians.* Anderson BJ, Rubin RR, Eds. Alexandria, VA, American Diabetes Association, 2002, p. 3–12

Anderson RM, Funnell MM, Arnold MS, Barr PA, Edwards GJ, Fitzgerald JT: Accessing the cultural relevance of an education program for urban African Americans with diabetes. *Diabetes Educ* 26:280–289, 2000

Anderson RM, Herman WH, Davis JM, Freedman RP, Funnell MM, Neighbors HW: Barriers to improving diabetes care for blacks. *Diabetes Care* 14:605–609, 1991

Arnold MS, Butler PM, Anderson RM, Funnell MM, Feste C: Guidelines for facilitating a patient empowerment program. *Diabetes Educ* 21:308–312, 1995

Aubert RE, Herman WH, Waters J, et al.: Nurse case management to improve glycemic control in diabetic patients in a health maintenance organization. *Ann Intern Med* 129:605–612, 1998

Bastable SB: *Nurse as Educator.* 2nd ed. Sudbury, MA, Jones and Bartlett, 2003

Becker MH, Janz NK: The health belief model applied to understanding diabetes regimen compliance. *Diabetes Educ* 11:41–47, 1985

Berkowitz KJ, Anderson LA, Panayioto RM, Zeimer DC, Gallina DL: Mini-residency on diabetes care for healthcare providers: enhanced knowledge and attitudes with unexpected challenges to assessing behavior change. *Diabetes Educ* 24:143–150, 1998

Biermann J, Toohey B: *The Diabetic's Total Health Book.* Los Angeles, Tarcher, 1980

Bonwell C, Eison J: *Active Learning: Creating Excitement in the Classroom.* Washington, DC, ERIC Clearinghouse on Higher Education, George Washington University, School of Education and Human Development, 1991

Brackenridge BP, Rubin RR: *Sweet Kids: How to Balance Diabetes Control and Good Nutrition with Family Peace.* Alexandria, VA, American Diabetes Association, 2002

Brackenridge B, Swenson K: Am I toast or is it just hot out here? Lessons from the desert in avoiding diabetes provider burnout. *Diabetes Spectrum* 12:23–28, 1999

Brown GC, Brown MM, Sharma S, Brown H, Gozum M, Denton P: Quality of life associated with diabetes mellitus in an adult population. *J Diabetes Complications* 14:18–24, 2000

Brown SA: Diabetes interventions for minority populations: "We're really not that different, you and I." *Diabetes Spectrum* 1:145–149, 1998

Carter JS, Pugh JA, Monterrosa A: Non-insulin-dependent diabetes mellitus in minorities in the United States. *Ann Intern Med* 125:221–232, 1996

Centers for Disease Control and Prevention: *National Diabetes Fact Sheet.* Atlanta, GA, US Department of Health and Human Services, Centers for Disease Control and Prevention, Division of Diabetes Translation, 1998

Charman D: Burnout and diabetes: reflections from working with educators and patients. *J Clin Psychol* 56:607–617, 2000

Close A: Patient education: a literature review. *J Adv Nursing* 13:203–213, 1998

Cohen SA: Patient education: a review of the literature. *J Adv Nursing* 6:11–18, 1981

Diabetes Control and Complications Trial Research Group: The effect of intensive treatment of diabetes on the development and progression of long-term complications in insulin-dependent diabetes mellitus. *N Engl J Med* 329:977–986, 1993

Drucker P: *The Leader of the Future*. San Francisco, CA, Jossey-Bass, 1996

Edelman SV: *Taking Control of Your Diabetes*. Cado, OK, Professional Communications, 2000

Fain JA, D'Eramo-Melkus G: Diabetes mellitus in young and middle adulthood. In *Management of Diabetes Mellitus: Perspectives of Care Across the Life Span*. 2nd ed. Haire-Joshu D, Ed. St. Louis, MO, Mosby, 1996, p. 729–754

Fast J: *Body Language*. New York, Pocket Books, 1975

Feste C: *The Physician Within: A Step-By-Step Guide to the Motivation You Need to Meet Any Health Challenge*. 2nd ed. New York, Henry Holt, 1995

Franz MJ, Monk A, Barry B, et al.: Effectiveness of medical nutrition therapy provided by dietitians in the management of non-insulin-dependent diabetes mellitus: a randomized, controlled trial. *J Am Diet Assoc* 95:1009–1017, 1995

Funnell MM: Lessons learned as a diabetes educator. *Diabetes Spectrum* 13:69–70, 2000

Funnell MM, Anderson RM: Putting Humpty Dumpty back together again: reintegrating the clinical and behavioral components in diabetes care and education. *Diabetes Spectrum* 12:19–23, 1999

Funnell MM, Donnelly MB, Anderson RM, Johnson PD, Oh MS: Perceived effectiveness, cost and availability of patient education methods and materials. *Diabetes Educ* 18:139–145, 1992

Funnell MM, Haas LB: National standards for diabetes self-management education programs: a technical review. *Diabetes Care* 18:100–116, 1995

Galanti GA: *Caring for Patients from Different Cultures*. Philadelphia, PA, University of Pennsylvania Press, 1991

Glasgow RE: Evaluating diabetes education. *Diabetes Care* 15:1423–1432, 1992

Glasgow RE: Outcomes of and for diabetes education research. *Diabetes Educ* 25 (Suppl.):74–88, 1999

Glasgow RE, Fisher EB, Anderson BJ, LaGreca A, Marrero D, Johnson SB, Rubin RR, Cox DJ: Behavioral science in diabetes: contributions and opportunities. *Diabetes Care* 22:832–843, 1999

Greenfield S, Kaplan SH, Ware JE Jr., et al.: Patient's participation in medical care: effects on blood sugar control and quality of life in diabetes. *J Gen Intern Med* 3:448–457, 1988

Grey M: Coping with diabetes. *Diabetes Spectrum* 13:167–169, 2000

Gronlund NE: *Measurement and Evaluation in Teaching.* 6th ed. New York, MacMillan, 1990

Grossman HY, Brink S, Hauser S: Self-efficacy in adolescent girls and boys with insulin-dependent diabetes mellitus. *Diabetes Care* 10:324–329, 1987

Haggard A: *Handbook of Patient Education.* Rockville, MD, Aspen, 1989

Hampson SE, Glasgow RE, Foster LE: Personal model of diabetes among older adults: relationship to self-management and other variables. *Diabetes Educ* 21:300–307, 1995

Healthcare Education Association: *Managing Hospital Education.* Laguna Niguel, CA, Healthcare Education Association, 1985

Health Care Financing Administration: Medicare program: expanded coverage for outpatient diabetes self-management training and diabetes measurements. *Federal Register* December 29, 2000

Health Literacy Network: Information on the Internet at *www.health literacy.net.* Accessed April 2001

Heins JM, Nord WR, Cameron M: Establishing and sustaining state-of-the-art diabetes education programs: research and recommendations. *Diabetes Educ* 18:501–508, 1992

Honan S, Krsnak G, Petersen D, Torkelson R: The nurse as patient educator: perceived responsibilities and factors enhancing role development. *J Contin Educ Nurs* 19:33–37, 1988

Houston C, Haire-Joshu D: Application of health behavior models to promote behavior change. In *Management of Diabetes Mellitus: Perspectives of Care Across the Life Span.* 2nd ed. Haire-Joshu D, Ed. St. Louis, MO, Mosby, 1996, p. 527–552

Janz NK, Becker MH: The health belief model: a decade later. *J Health Educ* 11:1–47, 1984

Johnson JA: Self-efficacy theory as a frame-work for community pharmacy-based diabetes education programs. *Diabetes Educ* 22:237–241, 1996

Joint Commission of Accreditation of Health Care Organizations: *Framework for Improving Performance.* Oakbrook Terrace, IL, Joint Commission of Accreditation of Health Care Organizations, 1994

Juran JM: *Juran's Quality Control Handbook.* 4th ed. New York, McGraw-Hill, 1998

Kort M: Motivation: the challenge for today's health promoter. *Can J Diabetes* 83:16–18, 1987

Kruger S: The patient educator role in nursing. *Appl Nurs Res* 1:19–24, 1991

Latter S, Clark JM, Wilson-Barnett J, Maben J: Health education in nursing: perceptions of practice in acute settings. *J Adv Nurs* 17:165–172, 1992

Lewis DJ, Saydak SJ, Mierzwa IP, Robinson JA: Gaming: a teaching strategy for adult learners. *J Contin Educ Nurs* 20:80–84, 1989

Lloyd CE, Dyer PH, Lancashire RJ, Harris T, Daniels JE, Barnett AH: Association between stress and glycemic control in adults with type 1 (insulin-dependent) diabetes. *Diabetes Care* 22:1278–1283, 1999

Lorenz RA, Bubb J, Davis D, et al.: Changing behavior: practical lessons from the Diabetes Control and Complications Trial. *Diabetes Care* 19:648–652, 1996

Lowe E, Arsham G: *Diabetes: A Guide to Living Well.* 3rd ed. Minneapolis, MN, Chronimed, 1997

Magenty J, Magenty M: Using self-efficacy theory in patient education. In *Managing Hospital-Based Patient Education.* Gilroth B, Ed. Chicago, IL, American Hospital Publishing, 1982, p. 327–337

Magenty J, Magenty M: *Patient Teaching.* Bowie, MD, Brady, 1982

Mager RF: *Preparing Instructional Objectives.* Belmont, CA, Fearon, 1975

Mangan M: Diabetes self-management education programs in the Veterans Health Administration. *Diabetes Educ* 23:687–695, 1997

McGoldrick TK, Jablonski RS, Wolf ZR: Needs assessment for a patient education program in a nursing department: a Delphi approach. *J Nurs Staff Dev* 10:123–130, 1994

McGinnis AL: *Bringing Out the Best in People.* Minneapolis, MN, Augsburg, 1985

McNabb WL, Quinn MT, Rosing L: Weight-loss program for inner-city black women with non-insulin-dependent diabetes mellitus: PATHWAYS. *J Am Diet Assoc* 93:75–77, 1993

Mulcahy K: Architects of the diabetes team. *Diabetes Educ* 25:161–162, 1999

Mulcahy KA, Peeples M, Tomky D, Weaver T, Upham P: National Diabetes Education Outcomes System: application to practice. *Diabetes Educ* 26:957–964, 2000

Murphy FG, Satterfield D, Anderson RM, Lyons AE: Diabetes educators as cultural translators. *Diabetes Educ* 19:113–116, 118, 1993

Narrow B: *Patient Teaching in Nursing Practice: A Patient- and Family-Centered Approach.* New York, Wiley, 1979

Nelson R, Wallick J: *Making Effective Presentations.* Glenville, IL, Scott, Forsman, 1990

Newstrom JW, Scannell EE: *Games Trainers Play.* New York, McGraw-Hill, 1980

Panno JM: A systematic approach for assessing learning needs. *J Nurs Staff Dev* 8:267–273, 1992

Peeples M, Mulcahy K, Tomky D, Weaver T: National Diabetes Education Outcomes System: a conceptual framework. *Diabetes Educ* 27:547–562, 2001

Peyrot M: Behavior change in diabetes education. *Diabetes Educ* 25 (Suppl. 6): 63–73, 1999

Peyrot M: Evaluation of patient education programs: how to do it and how to use it. *Diabetes Spectrum* 9:86–93, 1996

Peyrot M, Rubin RR: Living with diabetes: the patient-centered perspective. *Diabetes Spectrum* 7:204–205, 1994

Peyrot M, Rubin RR: Psychosocial aspect of diabetes care. In *Diabetes: Clinical Science in Practice.* Leslie D, Robbins D, Eds. Cambridge, Cambridge University Press, 1995, p. 465–477

Pichert JW, Smeltzer C, Snyder GM, Gregory RP, Smeltzer R, Kinzer CK: Traditional vs. anchored instruction for diabetes-related nutritional knowledge, skills, and behavior. *Diabetes Educ* 20:45–48, 1994

Piette JD: Interactive resources for patient education and support. *Diabetes Spectrum* 21:110–112, 2000

Pohl SL: Facilitating lifestyle change in people with diabetes mellitus: perspective from a private practice. *Diabetes Spectrum* 12:28–33, 1999

Poirier LM, Coburn KM: *Women & Diabetes: Staying Healthy in Body, Mind, and Spirit.* 2nd ed. Alexandria, VA, American Diabetes Association, 2000

Polonsky WH: Understanding and assessing diabetes-specific quality of life. *Diabetes Spectrum* 13:36–41, 2000

Polonsky WH, Welch GM: Listening to our patient's concerns: understanding and addressing diabetes-specific emotional distress. *Diabetes Spectrum* 9:8–11, 1999

Rankin SH, Stallings LD: *Patient Education: Issues, Principles and Practices.* 2nd ed. Philadelphia, PA, Lippincott, 1990

Raymond MW: Teaching toward compliance; a patient's perspective. *Diabetes Educ* 10:42–44, 1984

Rubin RR, Biermann J, Toohey B: *Psyching Out Diabetes: A Positive Approach to Your Negative Emotions.* 3rd ed. Los Angeles, Lowell, 1999

Rubin RR, Peyrot M: Quality of life and diabetes. *Diabetes Metab Res Rev* 15:205–218, 1999

Rubin RR, Peyrot M: Psychosocial problems and interventions in diabetes: a review of the literature. *Diabetes Care* 15:1640–1657, 1992

Rubin RR, Peyrot M, Saudek CD: Effect of diabetes education on self-care, metabolic control, and emotional well-being. *Diabetes Care* 12:673–679, 1989

Rubin RR, Peyrot M, Saudek CD: The effect of a diabetes education program incorporating coping skills training on emotional well-being and diabetes self-efficacy. *Diabetes Educ* 19:210–214, 1993

Ruggerio L: Helping people with diabetes change behavior: from theory to practice. *Diabetes Spectrum* 13:125–132, 2000

Ruggiero L, Prochaska JO: Introduction: readiness for change: application of the transtheoretical models to diabetes. *Diabetes Spectrum* 6:22–24, 1993

Shamoon H, Vaccaro-Olko MI: Diabetes education teams: professional education in diabetes. In *Proceedings of the DRTC Conference*. Bethesda, MD, National Diabetes Information Clearinghouse and National Institute of Diabetes and Digestive and Kidney Diseases, National Institutes of Health, 1980

Shillinger E: Locus of control: Implications for nursing practice. *Image J Nurs Sch* 15:58–63, 1983

Sims D, Sims E: From research to practice: motivation, adherence, and the therapeutic alliance. *Diabetes Spectrum* 2:49–51, 1989

Smith CE: Overview of patient education: opportunities and challenges for the twenty-first century. *Nurs Clin North Am* 24:583–587, 1989

Snoek FJ: Quality of life: a closer look at measuring patient's well-being. *Diabetes Spectrum* 3:24–28, 2000

Timms N, Lowes L: Autonomy or non-compliance in adolescent diabetes? *Br J Nurs* 8:794–800, 1999

Tomky D, Weaver T, Mulcahy K, Peeples M: Diabetes education outcomes: what educators are doing. *Diabetes Educ* 26:951–954, 2000

United Kingdom Prospective Diabetes Study Group: Effect of intensive blood-glucose control with metformin on complications in over-weight patients with type 2 diabetes (UKPDS 34). *Lancet* 352:854–865, 1998

U.S. Department of Health and Human Services, Office of Minority Health: Assuring cultural competence in health care: recommendations for national standards and outcomes-focused research agenda [article online], 2000. Available from *www.omhrc.gov/clas*. Accessed February 2001

Walker EA: Characteristics of the adult learner. *Diabetes Educ* 25 (Suppl. 6):16–24, 1999

Walker EA, Wylie-Rosett J, Shamoon H: Health education for diabetes self-management. In *Ellenberg and Rifin's Diabetes Mellitus*. 5th ed. Porte D Jr, Sherwin RS, Eds. Stamford, CT, Appleton & Lange, 1997

Wallhagen MI: Social support in diabetes. *Diabetes Spectrum* 12:254–256, 1999

Warshaw HS, Kulkarni K: *Complete Guide to Carb Counting*. Alexandria, VA, American Diabetes Association, 2001

Weaver T: Measuring outcomes: what, when, why, and how. *On the Cutting Edge: Diabetes Care and Education* 21:6–8, 2000

Weissberg-Benchell J, Pichert JW: Counseling techniques for clinicians and educators. *Diabetes Spectrum* 12:103–107, 1999

Williams GC, Freedman ZR, Deci EL: Supporting autonomy to motivate patients with diabetes for glucose control. *Diabetes Care* 21:1644–1651, 1998

About the American Diabetes Association

The American Diabetes Association is the nation's leading voluntary health organization supporting diabetes research, information, and advocacy. Its mission is to prevent and cure diabetes and to improve the lives of all people affected by diabetes. The American Diabetes Association is the leading publisher of comprehensive diabetes information. Its huge library of practical and authoritative books for people with diabetes covers every aspect of self-care—cooking and nutrition, fitness, weight control, medications, complications, emotional issues, and general self-care.

To order American Diabetes Association books: Call 1-800-232-6733. Or log on to http://store.diabetes.org

To join the American Diabetes Association: Call 1-800-806-7801. www.diabetes.org/membership

For more information about diabetes or ADA programs and services: Call 1-800-342-2383. E-mail: AskADA@diabetes.org or log on to www.diabetes.org

To locate an ADA/NCQA Recognized Provider of quality diabetes care in your area: www.ncqa.org/dprp

To find an ADA Recognized Education Program in your area: Call 1-888-232-0822. www.diabetes.org/recognition/education.asp

To join the fight to increase funding for diabetes research, end discrimination, and improve insurance coverage: Call 1-800-342-2383. www.diabetes.org/advocacy

To find out how you can get involved with the programs in your community: Call 1-800-342-2383. See below for program Web addresses.

- *American Diabetes Month:* Educational activities aimed at those diagnosed with diabetes—month of November. www.diabetes.org/ADM
- *American Diabetes Alert:* Annual public awareness campaign to find the undiagnosed—held the fourth Tuesday in March. www.diabetes.org/alert
- *The Diabetes Assistance & Resources Program (DAR):* Diabetes awareness program targeted to the Latino community. www.diabetes.org/DAR
- *African American Program:* Diabetes awareness program targeted to the African American community. www.diabetes.org/africanamerican
- *Awakening the Spirit: Pathways to Diabetes Prevention & Control:* Diabetes awareness program targeted to the Native American community. www.diabetes.org/awakening

To find out about an important research project regarding type 2 diabetes: www.diabetes.org/ada/research.asp

To obtain information on making a planned gift or charitable bequest: Call 1-888-700-7029. www.diabetes.org/ada/plan.asp

To make a donation or memorial contribution: Call 1-800-342-2383. www.diabetes.org/ada/cont.asp